YOGIC HOME EXERCISES

YOGIC HOME EXERCISES

EASY COURSE OF PHYSICAL CULTURE

FOR

MODERN MEN AND WOMEN

SWAMI SIVANANDA

GYAN

Published by

GYAN

Gyan Publishing House
5, Ansari Road
Daryaganj, New Delhi-110002
Phone: 011-47034999, 9811692060
E-mail: books@gyanbooks.com

Distribution Network
gyanbooks.com
India, USA, Canada, UK, Australia

ISBN: 978-93-6920-357-4 (HB)

First Published, 1944

2nd Impression 2025

Printed at: Gyan Press, Delhi.

YOGIC HOME EXERCISES
Author: SWAMI SIVANANDA

YOGIC HOME EXERCISES

OM

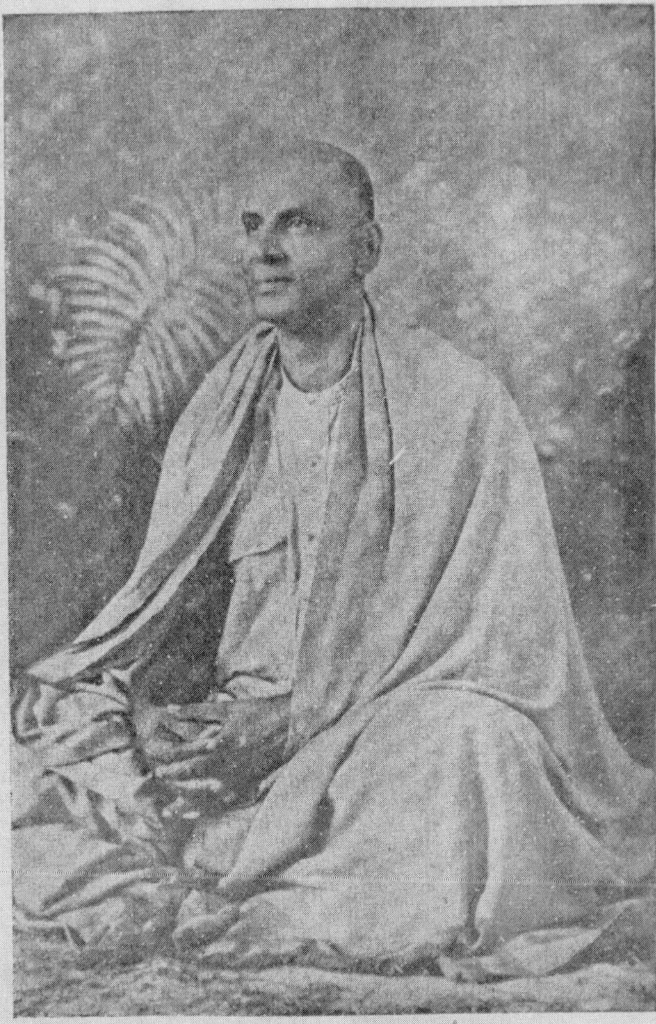

Sivamastu Sarvajagatam
Parahitanirata bhavantu bhut ganah
Doshah prayantu santim
Sarvatra sukhi bhavatu lokah

May there be welfare to the whole world; May all beings devote themselves to doing good to others; May all evils subside; May the world be happy in all ways!

SWAMI SIVANANDA
(*Frontispiece*)

Yogic Home Exercises

EASY COURSE OF PHYSICAL CULTURE

For

MODERN MEN AND WOMEN

By

SWAMI SIVANANDA

OM

DEDICATED

to men and women of
East and West who desire to
possess wonderful health, charming
and powerful personality and longevity,
abundant energy, muscular strength
and nerve-vigour through
the practice of
Yogic Exercises

OM

OM

UNIVERSAL PRAYER

Thou art, O Lord! the Creator of this Universe. Thou art the Protector of this world. Thou art in the Grass and the Rose. Thou art in the Sun and the Stars. Salutations unto Thee, O Destroyer of the cycle of Births and Deaths! Salutations unto Thee, O Bestower of Bliss and Immortality!

O Sweet Lord! May I be free from the bonds of Death. May I never again forget my Immortal nature! May I be able to look upon all beings with the equal vision! May I attain the supreme seat of Brahman! May I be free from impurity and sin! May I know my real essential nature!

Adorations to the Supreme Being, Who dwells in the hearts of all beings, Who is in the fire and water, Who is in the plants, herbs and trees, Who is in the stone, brick and iron bars, and Who has pervaded the whole universe.

I bow to Thee, O Secret of Secrets! I bow to Thee, O Indweller of hearts! I bow to Thee, O Silent Witness of all activities of all minds! I bow to Thee, O Inner Ruler of all beings, Who pervades and permeates and interpenetrates all things of this universe.

Salutations to Thee, the Supreme Lord! Thou art without beginning and without end. Thou art the flower. Thou art the bee. Thou art woman. Thou art man. Thou art the sea. Thou art the waves. Thou art the old man tottering with a stick. Thou art the saint. Thou art the rogue.

Thou art Light Divine. Thou art Light of Knowledge. Thou art the dispeller of darkness. Thou art the Supreme Guru. Thou art beyond the reach of mind and speech. Thou art beyond any kind of limitation. Thou art the Over-Soul. Thou art the Self of this Universe.

Thou art the Self-Luminous. Thou art without parts, without actions, without limbs, without any taint or fault, without birth and death. Thou art our Father, Mother, Brother, Friend, Relative, Guru and sole Refuge. Thou art the embodiment of Peace, Bliss, Knowledge, Power, Strength and Beauty.

O All-merciful Lord! Through Thy Grace, may I realise Truth. May I always entertain sublime thoughts. May I realise myself as the Light Divine. May I serve humanity with Atma Bhava. May I be free from greed, lust, egoism, jealousy, hatred. May I behold the one sweet immortal Self in all beings. May I realise Brahman with pure understanding.

May that Light of Lights ever guide me! May He cleanse my mind of all impurities! May He inspire me! May He bestow on me Power, Courage and Strength! May He remove the veil in the mind! May He remove all obstacles in the Spiritual path! May He make my life happy and fruitful! I bow to Thee, O Lord of Lords, O God of Gods, O Deva of Devas, the Brahman of the Upanishads, the Support for Maya and Ishwara, the Supreme Bridge, to Immortality!

OM Santi! OM Santi!! OM Santi!!!

SWAMI SIVANANDA

PREFACE

Good health is your greatest asset. Without good health you can hardly expect success in any walk of life. Even for spiritual pursuits good health is the pre-requisite. Without good health you cannot penetrate into the hidden depths of the vast ocean of life within and attain the final beatitude of life. Without good health you cannot wage war against the turbulent senses and the boisterous mind.

Regular practice of Yogic exercises or Yoga Asans even for fifteen minutes a day will keep you quite fit and soon make you hale and hearty. You will have abundant energy, muscular strength and nerve power, a charming personality and will live long.

There are now-a-days many systems of physical exercises. Among all the systems Yogic exercises or Yoga Asans stand unrivalled. It is the most perfect system. The brain, the muscles, the nerves, all the different organs and the tissues are toned up and energised. All chronic diseases are rooted out. In this book I have given a description of important exercises that are suitable for both men and women. The technique and the benefits derived are given for each exercise in detail.

I have divided the book into two parts. The first part contains valuable lessons on the theoretical knowledge necessary for the maintenance of health and strength. An elementary knowledge of the structure of the human body given in the First Chapter will prove of great use to the Yogic students. The Second Chapter throws much light on such important subjects as sleep, bath, diet, fast, etc. The Third Chapter deals with Brahmacharya which is essential for the maintenance of good health and strength.

In the second part of the book, you will find a number of selected Asans, Mudra, Bandha, Kriya and Pranayam exercises by the practice of which a busy man of the world can derive maximum benefits for an all-round development of the body by devoting only fifteen minutes daily. The practice of these Yogic exercises will without doubt bestow immense physical, mental and spiritual benefits on the student.

The readers will find a mine of spiritual instructions in the Appendix. Simple lessons on how to attain the goal of life, to control the thoughts, to control the senses and to obtain the conquest of mind are given in the Appendix. Practise the Yogic Exercises, follow the spiritual lessons, possess physical, mental, intellectual and spiritual powers and strength, and attain the Goal of Life—the Highest Happiness, the Supreme Peace!

I offer my cordial thanks to Yogi Prem Chaitanya, Rikhikesh, expert in Yoga Asans and Yogic Kriyas, for his demonstration of Asans in a graceful and explicit manner and thus helping me in taking his photos. I tender my sincere thanks also to Messrs. Goyal Photo Co., Dehra Dun, for their special attention and careful work.

Last but not least I express my keen sense of gratitude to Messrs. D. B. Taraporevala Sons & Co., Ltd., who have undertaken the work of publishing this work and thus spreading the knowledge of Hindu Rishis of yore, far and wide.

May you all attain good health, long life, and a high standard of vigour and vitality through the practice of Yogic Exercises and the Blessings of Rishis!

Hari OM Tat Sat!

SWAMI SIVANANDA.

"Ananda Kutir,"
Rikhikesh Dt.
Dehra Dun, (Himalayas).

CONTENTS

PART FIRST

INTRODUCTION

CHAPTER I

THE SCIENCE OF BODY STRUCTURE

CHAPTER II

HEALTH AND HYGIENE

CHAPTER III

BRAHMACHARYA

PART SECOND

CHAPTER I

YOGIC EXERCISES

CHAPTER II

PRANAYAM

CHAPTER III

RELAXATION

APPENDIX

ILLUSTRATIONS

INTRODUCTION

1. HEALTH AND FREEDOM

The whole universe from the mighty sun to the tiniest atom is controlled by law. There is perfect order everywhere. The sun performs its duties quite regularly. It rises at the proper time and sets at the proper time. The stars and planets revolve in an orderly manner. They are governed by laws. There are laws in the mental plane. There are laws of physics, of astronomy, of mathematics. There are laws of hygiene and health which govern our own being. In the vast universe man alone is the breaker of laws and the violator of rules. He is the single example of lawlessness and discord. He wilfully disregards the laws of health, leads a life of dissipation and then wonders why he suffers from diseases and disharmony. He deliberately ignores the rules of hygiene and right living and then weeps when he is ailing from an incurable malady.

What is that precious thing that makes life worth living? It is health. Will you sing today the song of "*Sariram Adhyam Kalu Dharma Sadhanam*—Body is indeed the foremost essential thing for the attainment of the goal of human existence or in other words it is verily the first important means in the accomplishment of the object of human life." Charak Maharishi says in his Samhita (Charaka Samhita): "*Dharmartha kama mokshanam arogyam moolamuttamam. Rogastasya aphartara sreyaso jivitayacha*—Health is the best cause of virtue, wealth, desire and emancipation, and is the blessedness of life. Diseases are the destroyers of health." The laws for the preservation of health should receive your foremost and first consideration. The laws of health are the laws of nature. These cannot be violated with impunity. Those who neglect these laws become victims to incurable diseases and drag on a cheerless existence.

Sattwic ahara or good wholesome food, rich in vitamins or a well-balanced diet, systematic practice of Asans and Pranayam, right and simple living and right thinking are the important requisites for the preservation of health and the attainment of a high standard of vigour and vitality. These are the sublime principles on which the Rishis and Yogins of yore lived a long peaceful life. These are the important methods on which they based the system of Yoga to achieve perfection in health of body and mind. These are the support on which the sinking nation must fall back if it wishes to regain her lost glory and splendour.

The world needs good healthy mothers, healthy and strong boys and girls. What do we find in these days in India? India, the land which produced Bishma, Bhima, Arjuna, Drona, Aswattama, Kripa, Parashuram and countless other chivalrous warriors, the soil which contained numberless Rajput chiefs of undaunted intrepidity, unparalleled chivalry and matchless strength abounds now with effeminate impotent weaklings. Children beget children. The laws of health are ignored and neglected. The nation is suffering and dying. The world requires numberless brave, moral Adhyatmic soldiers who are equipped with the five virtues, viz., Ahimsa, Satyam, Asteya, Brahmacharya and Aparigraha. Those who possess health and strength, those who are endowed with the above five virtues, those who have knowledge of the Self they alone can secure real freedom for the world.

2. HEALTH AND STRENGTH

Health is wealth. Health is a covetable possession indeed. Good health is a valuable asset for one and all. You should have physical as well as mental health. If you do not possess good health you cannot prosper in any walk of life.

Health is that state in which a man sleeps well, digests his food well, is quite at ease, is free from any kind of disease or uneasiness. When you are in a state of perfect health all the organs, viz., heart, lungs, brain, kidneys, liver, intestines work in perfect harmony and concord and discharge their functions satisfactorily. The pulse rate and the rate of respiration are in perfect order. The bodily temperature is normal. A healthy man smiles and laughs. He is cheerful and happy. He discharges his daily duties with ease and comfort. A healthy man is capable of doing work for a long time without getting fatigued. His bowels move very freely everyday. He possesses the highest kind of mental and physical efficiency.

A healthy man need not necessarily be strong and a strong man may not be healthy. A very strong man may suffer from many diseases. A healthy and strong man becomes a centre of great attraction. He radiates health and strength to all with whom he comes in contact.

By drinking pure water, by eating pure and wholesome food, by observing carefully the laws of health and hygiene, by taking regular exercise and cold baths in the morning, by practising Japa and meditation, by right living, right thinking, right action, right conduct, by observing Brahmacharya, by living in the open air and sunshine for some time daily, you can have wonderful health, vigour and vitality.

Strength and size are not always the same. Either a thin or wiry or a heavy-built man may be strong. Besides muscular strength you must have nerve strength as well. There are different kinds of strength. Some can lift heavy weights. Some can run a long distance quickly. Some can jump higher than others. Some can bear heat and cold better. Others can fast for days together without ill-effects. Some can bear any amount of pain. Some can bear insult and injury. Some can stop a car and break chains. Some can swim for a long distance. Others have great physical strength but they may not have mental strength. One harsh word can upset their balance of mind. Some people who have immense physical strength cannot bear the pain of an acute disease. They cry like children when they suffer from any disease. They have no mental strength. Some are afraid of public criticisms even though they may be physically strong.

He who possesses physical, mental, moral and spiritual strength is an ideal man. Moral strength is superior to physical strength. It is difficult to possess moral strength. Spiritual power is the highest power on earth. A Saint or a Yogi who possesses spiritual strength can move the whole world. He is a dynamic personality. The strength of Gandhiji was moral strength. He had gained the strength by the practice of Ahimsa, Satyam and Brahmacharya. Gandhiji had no physical strength. He had mental and moral strength. A powerful spiritual soul may dwell in a thin wiry body.

3. PHYSICAL AND MENTAL EFFICIENCY THROUGH YOGA

Every human being has within himself various potentialities and capacities of which he may never really have any conception. He is a magazine of power and knowledge. As he evolves he unfolds new powers, new faculties, new qualities.

Now he can change his environments. He can influence others. He can subdue other minds. He can heal others. He can get plenty of material things. He can conquer internal and external nature. He must awaken these dormant powers and faculties through the practice of Yoga. He must develop his will and control the senses and mind. He must purify himself. He must practise regular concentration. Then he will become a super-man or God-man.

Yoga is a perfectly practical system of self-culture. You can attain harmonious development of your body, mind, intellect and soul by the practice of Yoga. It is an exact science. This work deals with a system of Yogic exercises of the Indian Rishis and Yogins of yore based on exact principles. There is no vague doctrine here. It imparts to every practitioner definite practical knowledge, fine health, longevity, strength, vim and vitality. You can acquire absolute control over the whole of nature by the practice of Yoga. It will help you to attain ethical perfection, perfect concentration of the mind and to unfold various psychic powers. Yoga brings a message of hope to the forlorn, joy to the depressed, strength to the weak and knowledge to the ignorant. Yoga is the secret master-key that unlocks the realm of elysian bliss and deep abiding peace.

A Yogi or a Sage always keeps a balanced mind in all conditions of life and at all moments. A Yogi's vision is deeply penetrating because he has gathered all the dissipated rays of the mind by discipline through patient Sadhan. He can get full knowledge of either a distant or an internal object in no time. His mind is like a searchlight. Just as the diver in the pearl fishery dives down deep and brings up the pearl so also the mind of a Yogi dives deep into an object and brings out its truth in a moment. If the magnet is very powerful, it will influence iron filings even when they are placed at a long distance. Even so if the Yogi is an advanced person, he will have great influence over the people with whom he comes in contact. He can even exert his influence on persons living in a distant place.

Those who practise concentration evolve quickly. They can do any work with scientific accuracy. What others take six hours to do can be done by one who has concentration within half an hour. What others can read within six hours can be read by one who practises concentration within half an hour. Concentration purifies and calms the surging emotions, strengthens the current of thought and clarifies the ideas. Concentration helps a man in his material progress also. The man who practises concentration will have a very good outturn of work in his office or business house. What was cloudy and hazy before becomes clear and definite. What was difficult before becomes easy now and what was complex, bewildering and confusing before comes easily within the mental grasp. You can achieve anything through concentration. Nothing is impossible for one who practises concentration regularly. He who practises concentration will possess very good health and very clear mental vision.

The practice of Pranayama has a wonderful influence over the body, mind, intellect and the senses. It removes the diseases of the body and thoroughly renovates the cells and nerves. It supplies an abundance of fresh energy. It steadies the mind. It removes the impurities of the mind also. It strengthens the intellect and augments the intellectual capacities. It increases the power of memory. It calms the turbulent senses. It checks their outgoing tendencies. It bestows Nadi Shuddi (purification of the Nadis).

The lungs can be developed through the practice of deep breathing exercises. By the practice of Pranayama, the apices of the lungs will get the proper supply of oxygen. So they cannot harbour the germs of tuberculosis. The blood also will be pure. There will be an improvement in the quality and quantity of the blood. All the tissues and cells will be nourished with plenty of pure blood and lymph. The process of metabolism will be carried out in an efficient manner.

If the lungs are not developed properly they cannot perform the function of oxygenating the blood in an efficient manner. They will harbour readily the germs of consumption. You should try to possess a high lung power by the practice of Pranayama or deep breathing exercises. Lungs which are endowed with a good capacity, perform their functions satisfactorily under all conditions. They are proof against disease. In the vast majority of persons breathing is shallow and without rhythm. Lungs which have a good reserve capacity achieved by the practice of Pranayama and deep breathing exercises will turn out extra work when there is an extra demand made upon them on account of lowered vitality from some cause or other. Pranayama or deep breathing exercises invigorate the nerves, energise the heart and the circulation of blood, improve digestion, augment the vital force and help the liver to perform its work efficiently.

The practice of Asans develops the body and the practitioner is agile and nimble. He has a very elastic spine and supple body. He has a keen vigorous appetite. Any trouble is removed from its starting point by the practice of Asans. The three important organs, viz., heart, lungs and brain and the cerebro-spinal system are kept in a healthy condition by a regular practice of Asans. The vital forces are also preserved and increased. The circulation of blood in the arteries and veins is kept in proper order by the practice of Asans. There is no stagnation of blood in any part of the body. The spinal cord is toned up. The practice of Asans prevents the development of arteriosclerosis or hardening of the arteries. The practice of Asans, in fact, lubricates the whole bodily system.

Abundant blood is supplied to the brain by the practice of Sirshasan. Hence the memory and intellectual powers are increased. The practitioner regains his memory power that may have been lost owing to overwork or some other causes. It transmutes the sex-energy into spiritual power or Ojas Shakti. The nerves of the body are energised and galvanised.

The practitioner always laughs heartily and radiates joy, strength and vigour wherever he moves. He always accomplishes his aims. He always gets success in all his attempts. He looks very young even at the age of sixty. He is endowed with a peculiar glow in his face and eyes and possesses a peculiar charm in his smile. By practising the Asans regularly, men and women will acquire a figure which will enhance their beauty and that suppleness which gives charm and elegance to every movement.

Now you must clearly understand that you can attain physical and mental efficiency through Yoga. Destroy all weakness by regular and systematic practice of it. Attain harmonious development of your body, mind, intellect and soul by a regular practice of Yoga. Health is thy birthright but not disease. Strength is thy heritage but not weakness; efficiency but not inefficiency; courage but not fear; bliss but not sorrow; peace but not restlessness; knowledge but not ignorance; immortality but not mortality. Attain this birthright or Divine heritage and shine as a fully developed Yogi radiating Joy, Peace, Bliss and Knowledge everywhere !

4. THE BENEFITS OF YOGIC EXERCISES

This body is the moving temple of God. It is an instrument for crossing the ocean of Samsar or the round of births and deaths and attaining the supreme abode of immortality, eternal bliss and perennial joy. It is a horse that can take you to the destination or the goal of life. Therefore it must be kept quite healthy and strong. Proper training and care of the body on an intelligent basis is necessary. There should be a harmonious development of all the muscles of the body, organs, nerves, and the frame.

Some try to develop the chest and the arms only. Some try to develop only the lower limbs and the chest. To develop certain parts of the body at the expense of the rest of the body is irrational and unscientific. Another important point is, there must not be any violent exertion. The general health must be maintained. There must be symmetrical development of all the parts of the body. The muscles of the extremities or limbs, chest, back, neck, abdomen, etc., should be developed equally. Then only will there be grace, elegance and beauty. You should have a comprehensive understanding of the laws of health and hygiene and dietetics, of the causes of ill-health, how they arise, how they may be prevented or removed! An elementary knowledge of physiology which treats of the functions of the human body and anatomy which treats of the structure of the body will be of immense help to you.

This is a system of Yogic exercises of the Indian Rishis and Yogins of yore based on exact principles. There is no vague doctrine here. It imparts to every practitioner definite, practical knowledge, fine health, longevity, strength, vim and vitality. Any trouble is removed from its starting point by the practice of Asans. These are adapted for both men and women, for people of the East and West. You can keep up meditation while performing the Asans. This is accompanied by Pranayam or regulation of breath also. By practising the Asans regularly men and women will acquire a figure which will enhance their beauty and that suppleness which will give charm and elegance to every movement of theirs.

These Yogic exercises are preventive and curative. That is the beauty of this system. Some exercises twist the body forward and backward. Others help the lateral movement of the spine. Thus the body as a whole is developed, toned up and strengthened. The whole course can be finished in fifteen minutes. Within this short period you can realise the maximum benefit. All the organs of the body are toned up and exercised. This system is simple, exact, efficacious, economical of time and capable of being self-practised.

Abundant blood is supplied to the brain by the practice of Sirshasan. Hence the memory and intellectual powers are increased. The practitioner regains his memory power that may have been lost owing to overwork or other causes. The spinal nerve-roots and the spinal cord receive an abundant supply of blood. Eyesight improves by the practice of Sirshasan. Grey hairs also disappear. Many incurable diseases are cured by the regular practice of this Asan. Wet-dreams are checked. It transmutes the sex-energy into spiritual power or Ojas Shakti. The nerves of the body are energised, invigorated and galvanised.

The endocrine glands play an important part in the economy of nature. The practice of Sarvangasan keeps the thyroid in a healthy condition. A healthy thyroid means healthy functioning of all the organs and systems of the body. The suprarenals or the adrenals, the pituitary and the pineal glands are also toned up and maintained in a healthy condition.

The diaphragm, the muscular partition between the chest and the abdomen is also developed by certain exercises such as Dhanurasan, Mayurasan, Paschimottanasan. The movements of the diaphragm massage the abdominal viscera or organs. There will be free evacuation of the bowels daily in the morning. Constipation, dyspepsia and a host of other ailments of the stomach and the intestines will be eradicated.

For those who have a poorly-developed chest, respiratory exercises are necessary. For those who have excess of fat in the abdomen, abdominal exercises are essential. They should pay special attention to them. Exercises that are best calculated to improve the function of the vital inner organs of the body and tone them up to counteract against their tendency to disease, are also indispensably requisite. Then only a high standard of health, vigour and vitality will be maintained.

The lungs can be developed through the practice of deep breathing exercises. By Pranayam, the apices of the lungs will get a proper supply of oxygen. There will be an improvement in quality and quantity of the blood. All the tissues and cells will be nourished with plenty of pure blood and lymph. The process of metabolism will be carried out in an efficient manner.

The circulation of blood in the arteries and veins is kept in proper order by the practice of Asans. There is no stagnation of blood in any part of the body. The spinal cord is toned up. The practice of Asans prevents arteriosclerosis or hardening of the arteries. The practitioner remains for ever agile and nimble. He has a very elastic spine and a supple body. He has a keen vigorous appetite.

If the joints move freely, the ligaments and the surrounding tissues will be in a properly healthy condition. Free movement of the spine will prevent stiffening and contraction of the spine. Ossification and degeneration of the bones of the spinal column (Meru Danda) will also be checked. A thickened and immovable joint due to lack of free movement gives a great deal of discomfort and uneasiness. By the practice of Asans free movement is given to the elbow, wrist, ankle, shoulder and spinal joints. Muscles of the cervical, dorsal and lumbar regions are stretched and relaxed. There is dorsal and lumbar lifting, through frame exercises. The body is kept in a fit condition.

If the muscles are not properly exercised, they will contract. The blood circulation and nerve force will consequently be impeded. Then functional disturbances of the organs and general nerve-tone will result. The muscles will get atrophied. Practice of Asans keeps the muscles, organs and nerves in a very healthy condition.

Sound functioning of the organs, depends upon good healthy nerves. The tripods of life are the brain, the heart and the lungs. The heart and the lungs are under the control of the brain. The heart and the lungs and the other organs are stimulated or retarded through nerves that proceed from the brain and the spinal cord. These three important organs and the cerebro-spinal system are kept in a healthy condition by a regular practice of Asans. The vital forces are also preserved and increased.

Therefore this is the perfect system of physical culture. This is the king of all systems of physical culture. This is the best of all systems of exercises. Practise these Yogic exercises and have a strong healthy body. There is no use in theorising. What is wanted is regular, systematic, sustained practice. An ounce of practice is better than tons of theory. Regularity in the practice is very necessary. Many people practise these exercises by fits and starts and give up the practice after some months and hence they do not derive the maximum benefits of this system of exercises. He who practises regularly will be endowed with a peculiar glow in his face and eyes and a peculiar charm in his smile. He will always laugh heartily and radiate joy, strength and vigour wherever he moves. He will accomplish all his cherished aims. He will always succeed in all his attempts. He will look very young even at the age of sixty.

CHAPTER I

The Science of Body Structure

1. BODY AND MIND

The mind is intimately connected with the body. The body helps the mind and the mind helps the body. The health of mind and the body are undoubtedly bound up in each other. The mind acts upon the body and the body reacts upon the mind. If the body is sick, the mind also becomes sick. If the body is strong and healthy, the mind also becomes healthy and strong. Understand the nature of the mind and keep it in a very healthy condition. Be always cheerful. Cheerfulness is the best mental tonic.

The mind has a great influence over the whole body. Grief in the mind weakens the body. Body influences the mind also in its turn. A healthy body makes the mind healthy. A pain in the stomach causes a mental depression. The body is the shadow of the mind. It is a mould prepared by the mind into which it pours forth its energies. A pure mind means a healthy body.

When the mind is agitated then the body also is agitated. Wherever the body goes, the mind follows. When the body and the mind are agitated, the Prana flows in a wrong direction. Instead of pervading the whole body steadily and equally, it will vibrate at an unequal rate (unrhythmically). Then, food is not digested properly. Diseases originate. If the primary cause be removed then all diseases will soon disappear.

2. THE SKELETON

A mason builds a house out of stones, small bricks, chunam (lime) and cement. He uses big pieces of stones for the construction of the main walls and puts small bricks and pebbles to fill up the crevices in the walls, plasters the walls with chunam and eventually puts a layer of cement. He polishes the walls with finishing touches and gives a colouring in the end to attract the eye. Even so the Divine Architect, Ishwar, has constructed this human body with the help of Mother Prakriti. The bones represent the big stones; the muscles represent the pebbles; the fat the bricks; the dermis or white skin is comparable to chunam; the skin or epidermis to the cement; the pigment of the skin to the colouring matter. Look at the marvellous skill of the Divine Engineer, the Engineer of engineers! The muscles are fixed to the bones by means of tendons. The joints are kept intact by ligaments. Deposition of fat gives good shape to the limbs, the trunk and the abdomen and gives beauty to the body.

The bones are the principal organs of support, and the passive instruments of locomotion. Connected together in the skeleton, they form a framework of hard material, affording attachment to the soft parts, maintaining them in their due position, sheltering such as are of delicate structure, giving stability to the whole fabric, and preserving its shape. The entire skeleton in the adult consists of about two hundred distinct bones. They are distributed as follows:

Cranium	8
Face	14
Hyoid	1
The spine (sacrum and coccyx included)	26
Sternum and ribs	26
Upper extremities	64
Lower extremities	62
Total	201

In this enumeration the Patellae or knee-pans or knee-caps are included as separate bones, but the smaller Sesamoid (shaped like sesame seed) bones consisting of several small bones which are found embedded in tendons covering the bones of the knees, hand and foot bones and the small bones of the middle ear, viz., Malleus 2, Incus 2, and Stapes 2, are not included.

(a) Spine

The spine is also known as the vertebral column. In Sanskrit it is called Meru Danda. It is made up of a row of bones called vertebrae. It is about twenty-eight inches long in a man of average height and reaches from the hips to the head. The bodies of the vertebrae are piled one upon another forming a solid, strong pillar for the support of the head and trunk. The neck spine contains seven bones. The chest spine contains twelve bones. The waist contains five bones. The hips contain five bones. The tail contains four bones. There is a tunnel or tube in the centre of the column along which passes the spinal cord which takes its origin from the brain. From between each pair of spine bones small bundles of nerves pass out on either side to reach the different parts of the body which they control.

The spine can be bent forwards or backwards or to either side. It can be turned also from its middle position to one side or the other. The different parts of the spine are capable of differing amounts of movement. The chest spine moves less than the waist spine in bending backward. The amount of motion permitted is the greatest in the region of the neck. Care of the spine is very necessary. It is a very important structure as it shelters main groups of nerves. You must keep it healthy, strong and supple by bending and stretching it in all directions—forwards and backwards, to one side and the other and by twisting it round as far as it will go once every day. Whenever a movement is limited, the circulation of blood to that part of the body is slower and smaller. Consequently the joints and muscles are not properly nourished. They are not also properly cleansed of their waste products. If the spine is supple, then alone will you be able to hold it straight.

(b) Chest

The thorax or chest cavity is an elongated bony cage. The chest contains the most important organs—the heart and the lungs. There are two lungs, the right lung and the left lung. The heart is placed between the two lungs. The lungs and the heart are important not only for health but for life itself. It behoves therefore that you should have as good a chest as possible.

The chest has walls and a floor. The walls are formed by a part of the spine, usually 12 of its bones, to which are attached 12 ribs on each side. The first seven ribs are joined to the breast-bone, sternum, by bands of cartilage. The next three are attached to the band of the seventh. The ends of the last two float more freely in the muscles. They are called floating ribs. The floor of the chest cavity is formed by the diaphragm or dome-shaped midriff.

(c) Abdomen

The adbomen extends from the tip of the breast bone or sternum right down to the hips. The pelvis also is a portion of the abdominal cavity. Its top is the dome-shaped diaphragm. Its walls are formed partly of bones and partly of muscles. Inside the abdomen are located many vital organs. The stomach lies close under the left side of the diaphragm. On the right side is the liver. Below these two lie the intestines in a long and twisted course. Low down in the front is the bladder. Behind are two kidneys. Good abdominal movements mean good digestion and circulation and more effective excretion.

(d) Legs and Arms

The arm has a single bone known as the Humerus. The forearm is made up of two bones, viz., Radius and Ulna. The Radius is on the outer side and the Ulna is on the inner side of the forearm. The thigh has one bone, Femur. The leg is made up of two bones like the forearm, viz., Tibia on the inner side and Fibula on the outer side. The legs are in some ways similar to the arms. The hip bones and the shoulder blades both have a socket or hollow in which moves the rounded head of the single bones of the upper part of the limbs. The sockets or hollows on the hip bone are very deep. Into them fit the rounded heads of the thigh bones. The socket of the shoulder-blade is very shallow. The feet with five toes and the hands and a thumb are similar in their arrangement. Legs bear the weight of the body. Their movements are neither so fine nor so varied as those of the arms. The shoulder-blades move in many directions but the hip bones are fixed on to the spine. Your whole carriage is built on your feet.

3. MUSCLES

The muscles are fastened to the bones by means of ligaments and tendons. You must correct the faults which your habitual positions cause in your muscles and make the short longer and the long shorter. If you do not use a muscle it will become smaller. If you use it very much it will grow larger. You can develop all the muscles by suitable exercises. "Loosening exercises," such as shaking, vibration, swinging, make the muscles loose and supple. These exercises eliminate from the joints and muscular tissues the waste products that induce fatigue.

A muscle becomes shorter when it receives a nerve-message. When a muscle which is fastened on the two bones becomes shorter, it pulls the bones towards each other Then the bones move. When the nerve stops sending the message the shortened muscle relaxes and the bones are pushed back to their original position. Another group of muscles do this part of the work.

(a) Muscles of the Back

The muscles of the back are disposed in five layers, one beneath the other. The two largest and most superficial muscles are: Trapezius and Latissimus dorsi. The trapezius is a very large muscle and covers the other muscles of the upper part of the back and neck, as well as the upper part of the latissimus dorsi. The latissimus dorsi muscles act upon the bones of the upper extremities. They elevate the shoulders, move the arms and assist in drawing up the body in climbing.

(b) Muscles of the Chest

The chief bulk of the anterior muscular wall of the chest is made up of the pectoral muscles, viz., Pectoralis major and Pectoralis minor. The Pectoralis minor is underneath and entirely covered by the Pectoralis major. These muscles move the arms.

(*c*) Muscles of the Thorax

The muscles of the thorax are chiefly concerned with the movements of the ribs during respiration. They are the intercostals and Levatores Costarum. The intercostals are found filling the spaces between the ribs. Each muscle consists of two layers, one external and one internal. There are eleven internal spaces on each side and two muscles on each space. Therefore there are 44 intercostal muscles. The fibres of these muscles run in opposite directions. The action of the external fibres is to pull the ribs upwards and outwards, thereby increasing the chest cavity. The action of the internal fibres is to depress the ribs. The Levatores Costarum muscles are the lifters of the ribs. They assist in elevation of the first ten ribs and with the other muscles draw the lower ribs backwards.

(*d*) Muscles of the Diaphragm

The diaphragm is a thin, musculo-fibrous partition between the thoracic and abdominal cavities. It is dome-shaped, and has three openings for the passage of Aorta, the large artery in the body, the inferior Vena Cava, one of the largest veins in the body and the oesophagus or gullet. The diaphragm is the great respiratory muscle of the body.

The mechanical act of respiration consists of two sets of movements, viz., those of inspiration and of expiration, in which air is successfully drawn into the lungs and expelled from them by the alternate increase and diminution of the thoracic cavity. In the act of inspiration the diaphragm contracts and in contracting flattens out and descends, the abdominal organs are pressed downwards, and the thorax is expanded vertically. The diaphragm is an expulsive as well as the chief respiratory muscle of the body.

(*e*) Muscles of the Abdomen

The muscular walls of the abdomen are mainly formed by three layers of muscles, the fibres of which run in different directions, those of the superficial and middle layers being oblique and those of the innermost layer being transverse. The chief muscles of the abdomen are external oblique, internal oblique, rectus abdominis and transversalis. Linea Alba or white line is a tendinous band formed by the union of the aponeuroses of the oblique and transverse muscles. It extends perpendicularly down the middle line from the sternum to the pubis.

The abdominal muscles compress the abdominal organs by constricting the cavity of the abdomen. They give assistance in expelling the foetus from the womb, the excreta or faeces from the rectum, the urine from the bladder and the contents of the stomach in vomitting. They are much assisted by the descent of the diaphragm. The abdominal muscles raise the diaphragm and assist in expiration. They draw the pelvis upwards as a preparatory step to the elevation of the lower limbs in the action of climbing.

(*f*) Muscles of the Upper Extremities (Upper Limbs)

The most prominent muscles found in the upper limbs are the Deltoid, Biceps, Triceps, Pronators, Supinators, Flexors and Extensors. The deltoid is a coarse triangular muscle that covers the top of the shoulder. It raises the arms from the sides so as to bring them at right angles to the trunk.

Biceps: This is a long fusiform muscle. It occupies the whole of the anterior surface of the arm. It is divided above into two portions or heads, hence the name biceps. It flexes the forearm on to the upper arm.

Triceps: This muscle is situated on the back of the arm. It is of a large size and divided above into three heads. Hence the name triceps. It is the extensor muscle of the forearm. It is the direct antagonist of the biceps. The extensor muscle is the one that helps in the extension of the limbs.

The muscles that cover the forearm are disposed in groups, the pronators and flexors being placed on the front and inner part of the forearm and the Supinators and Extensors on the outer side and back of the forearm. They are antagonistic to one another. The pronators turn the palm of the hand backward and when the elbow is flexed, downwards or prone. The supinators turn the palm of the hand forwards, and when the elbow is flexed, upwards or into the supine position. The flexors and extensors serve to flex and extend the wrist and fingers.

(*g*) Muscles of the Lower Extremities (Lower Limbs)

These include the muscles of the hip, thigh, leg and foot. The most important of these muscles are: Glutei or gluteai muscles, Psoas Magnus, Posterior Femoral, Anterior Femoral, Internal Femoral, Tibialis Interior, Extensors, Peroneal, Gestrocnemius, Soleus, Flexors, Tibialis Posterior.

If we compare the muscles of the shoulder, arm and forearm with those of the hip, the thigh and the leg, we shall see that the anterior muscles of the former correspond roughly with the posterior muscles of the latter and the muscles of the hip, thigh and leg are larger and coarser in texture than those of the shoulder, arm and forearm.

Glutei: Three gluteal muscles—Gluteus maximus, Gluteus medius and Gluteus minimus—form the chief prominence of the buttocks. The Gluteus medius and Gluteus minimus are under the Gluteus maximus. These muscles support the trunk upon the head of the femur and bring the body into the erect position when the trunk is bent forwards upon the thigh.

Psoas Magnus: This is the great loin muscle. Its action is flexion and external rotation of the thigh.

Posterior Femoral: Posterior femoral or the hamstring muscles cover the back of the thigh. There are three of these muscles—the biceps, the semitendinosus and the semimembranosus. The chief of these is the biceps, and is somewhat analogous to the biceps covering the front of the arm. The action of the hamstring muscles is to flex the knee and extend the thigh.

Anterior Femoral: The principal anterior femoral muscles are the Quadriceps and the Sartorius.

Quadriceps: This is a four-headed muscle that covers the front of the thigh, and is analogous to the triceps covering the back of the arm. Each head is described as a separate muscle: (1) Rectus Femoris, (2) Vastus Externus, (3) Vastus Internus, (4) Vastus Intermedius. The quadriceps is the great extensor of the leg. It also flexes the thigh and antagonises the action of the hamstring muscles.

Sartorius: This muscle, Sartorius, is often called the "Tailor's muscle." It is a long ribbon-like muscle. It is the longest in the body, and is the muscle principally concerned in producing the posture assumed by the tailor in sitting cross-legged and hence its name.

Internal Femoral: The internal femoral is otherwise known as adductor muscles. These muscles are also adductors of the thigh.

The Tibialis anterior, the extensors and the peroneal muscles cover the front and outer side of the leg. The Gastrocnemius and the Soleus, the Flexors and the Tibialis Posterior cover the back of the leg.

The action of the Tibialis anterior and one of the three peroneal muscles (Peroneus Tertius) is to flex the ankle, while the action of the Tibialis Posterior and the other Peroneal muscles (Peroneus Longus, Peroneus Brevis) is to extend the ankle. The flexors and extensors act on the toes.

The Gastrocnemius muscles form the calves of the legs. They possess considerable power, and are constantly in use while standing, walking, dancing or leaping.

4. MUSCLES AND NERVES

The function of the muscles is to contract so that their two ends are drawn together, and a movement is thus produced which by various systems of levers can be converted into the particular form of motion required. For example. the contraction of the muscles of the calf draws the heel upward, and in this way causes the whole body to be elevated on the toes.

In order to bring about a muscular contraction the muscle must first be stimulated. The way in which the muscle is normally stimulated is through its nerve, which conducts the nerve impulses from the central nervous system to the muscle fibres. Arriving at the latter, the nerve impulses bring about the complex chemical changes upon which the contraction of the muscle depends. When the nerve impulses cease, the muscle relaxes again.

5. BRAIN AND NERVES

The nervous system is a collection of nervous tissues set apart as a special apparatus for the reception and transmission of nerve-impulses. This apparatus consists of the brain, and the spinal cord which is attached to the brain. Many nerve trunks emerge from both and go to all parts of the body and eventually terminate in nerve-endings. The nerve-fibres are in connection with aggregations of nerve-tissue called nerve-ganglia. A ganglion is a small collection of cell-bodies connected by means of nerve-fibres and dendrites with other ganglia and with the central nervous system. The whole nervous system itself is made up of tiny microscopic elements called neurones.

The brain and the spinal cord constitute the central nervous system. The brain is placed in the cranial cavity. The spinal cord extends from the brain, runs along the vertebral canal of the vertebral bones or the spinal column. There are 31 pairs of spinal nerves.

The brain is the most complex and the largest mass of nervous tissues in the body. It is contained in the cranial cavity. It is made up of white and grey matter. It is divided into four principal parts, viz., the cerebrum, the cerebellum or "little brain," the pons varolii and the medulla oblongata.

The medulla oblongata is the seat of several important or vital centres. It contains the respiratory centres for regulating the functions of respiration; the cardiac centres which control the rate and force of the heart's action; the vasomotor centre to regulate the size of the small arteries or blood vessels in any part of the body at any particular time, thus controlling the amount of blood furnished to that part; other centres, such as the vomitting centre, heat controlling centre, etc. If the medulla is seriously injured, death will result immediately.

The cranial nerves, twelve in number on each side, arise from the base of the brain and medulla oblongata and pass out through openings in the base of the skull. They are (1) Olfactory (sensory); (2) Optic (sensory); (3) Oculo-motor (motor); (4) Trochlear (motor); (5) Trifacial or trigeminal (mixed, but mainly sensory); (6) Abducens (motor); (7) Facial (motor); (8) Auditory (sensory); (9) Glosso-pharyngeal (mixed); (10) Pneumogastric or vagus (mixed); (11) Spinal accessory (motor); (12) Hypoglossal (motor).

The olfactory is the special nerve of the sense of smell. The optic nerve is the special nerve of the sense of sight. The oculo-motor nerve supplies all the muscles of the eye except the superior oblique and external rectus. The trochlear nerve supplies only the superior oblique muscle of the eye. The trifacial is the largest of the cranial nerves. The opthalmic, the superior maxillary and the inferior maxillary are the three branches of the trifacial nerve. The abducens nerve supplies the external rectus muscle of the eye. The facial nerve is the motor nerve of all the muscles of expression in the face.

The auditory nerve is the special nerve of the sense of hearing. The glosso-pharyngeal nerve is distributed to the tongue and the pharynx being the nerve of sensation belonging to the mucous membrane of the pharynx, conveys motion to the muscles of the pharynx and is the special nerve of taste belonging to a part of the tongue.

The pneumogastric nerve has a more extensive distribution than any other cranial nerves. It passes through the neck and thorax to the upper part of the abdomen. It contains both motor and sensory fibres. It supplies the organs of voice production and respiration with motor and sensory filaments and the pharynx, oesophagus, stomach and heart with motor fibres (cardiac inhibitory).

The spinal accessory nerve consists of two parts, one the spinal portion and the other the accessory portion of the tenth nerve. It is a motor nerve. It supplies certain muscles of the neck, and arises from the spinal cord. The hypoglossal nerve is the motor nerve belonging to the tongue.

It will be observed that of the 12 pairs of cranial nerves, four and a part of the fifth are distributed to the eye, viz. the optic, motor oculi, trochlear, abducens and the opthalmic branch of the fifth. The ear has one special nerve, the auditory, and is sparingly supplied with motor and sensory fibres from other nerves. The nose also has one special nerve, the olfactory, and is more abundantly supplied than the ear with motor and sensory fibres from other nerves. The tongue has two special branch nerves of taste—the lingual, a branch of the fifth, and the glossal, a branch of the ninth; it has also its own motor nerve, the hypoglossal.

It is difficult to answer what the nature of the nerve impulse is. The nerve-fibre serves as a conveyor of nerve impulses. The speed at which an impulse travels along an efferent nerve-fibre is about 140 feet per second. An afferent impulse travels somewhat slower, 110 feet per second. Efferent nerves carry the nerve impulses from the nerve-cell to the nerve-endings, i.e., from the brain towards the skin. Those in which the impulses travel in the reverse direction from the skin towards the brain are called the afferent nerves. It is the afferent nerve that carries the sensation of pain from the finger to the brain when a scorpion stings the finger! It is the efferent nerve that carries the impulse from the brain towards the finger which makes us take the finger away from the scorpion. Everything is done in the fraction of a second. The afferent impulse goes to the spinal cord from the skin and from the spinal cord it is transmitted to the brain. The efferent impulse comes from the brain to the spinal cord and from the spinal cord it is transmitted to the skin. The spinal cord is thus the *via media* between the brain and the skin.

Other sets of nerves carry on the function of digestion, circulation, etc. They perform their work independently. You need not think about them at all. They go on with their work whether you are asleep or awake. These are the self-governing nerves that belong to the sympathetic nervous system. The sympathetic system sends motor impulses to the involuntary muscles, conveys sensations from the different organs, controls the vasomotor system, the heart's action and secretion.

The brain is divided into two halves by a fissure or groove in the middle. The left side of the brain transmits messages to the right side of the body and *vice versa*. The main nerves of the central nervous system control all voluntary movements of the body. Through the play of these nerves we move our limbs, walk, run, jump, etc. All the nerves are in direct communication with the sympathetic nervous system which controls the involuntary functions, such as digestion, circulation of blood, etc. The two nervous systems are inter-dependent. The sympathetic depends for its energy and efficient working on the central nervous system. The central nervous system is sustained and built up by the blood manufactured and circulated through the agency of the sympathetic. Lowering of vitality of the sympathetic system will react on the central nervous system.

The sympathetic system is made up of a chain of nerve fibres which run down each side of the spine. Just in front of it, there is a ganglion in each fibre. All these nerve fibres form the 'solar-plexus' which governs the functions of the digestive organs, the liver, kidneys, etc. If there is any disorder in the sympathetic system, ganglia or the 'solar-plexus' you will suffer from torpidity of the liver. The kidneys will not perform their function efficiently. You will experience some congestion here, a pain or irritation there, a little swelling in the feet or the cheeks, a little burning in the stomach and so on.

The sympathetic and the para-sympathetic constitutes the autonomic system which is to some extent independent of the central nervous system. The action of the sympathetic fibres is antagonistic to the action of the fibres of the para-sympathetic. The sympathetic nerves accelerate the heart's action, while the para-sympathetic system retards the action of the heart. The sympathetic chain is a system of a ganglia vertically arranged on both sides of the spinal column. The major part of the para-sympathetic system is made up by the vagus.

A Yogi can control the automatic nervous system. By suppressing all voluntary and involuntary actions he can bring the working of the human machine to a standstill. In the year 1926 under the auspices of the Bombay Medical Union, Desabandhu demonstrated certain Yogic feats, such as the stopping of the radial and the temporal pulse on both sides at will. He stopped the beatings of the heart for a few seconds. Through the practice of Kechari Mudra and Pranayama, Yogis have buried themselves for days and even months.

6. HEALTH AND HORMONES

Hormones are the products secreted by the endocrine glands. They are internal secretions. The endocrine glands are ductless glands which discharge their several products or internal secretions directly into the blood stream and thereby influence all the regions of the body. These secretions affect every function of the body both physiological and psychological.

These endocrine glands are small wonderful chemical factories which manufacture very potent substances called hormones. These hormones regulate the chemistry of our lives. They markedly influence our structure, our health and our whole personality.

The most important advance in Medical Science made during recent years is the discovery of the inner glands of the body and their importance to life. It has been proved that the glands control our entire life, energy, and mental and physical activity.

The body is a very intricate and complex machine. Hormone regulation is very important in the normal functioning of the human organism. Height, stature, the shape of the face, the appearance, intelligence, bodily development, the complexion, colour, and the characteristic differences between men and women, such as the temper, the voice, the growth of the hair, mental and physical capacity, the formation of the body and even the emotions are regulated by the functioning of these mysterious glands. Even the individual, radical characteristics of every man, woman and child are attributed to the varying amounts of hormones manufactured by the endocrine glands of their bodies.

How wonderful is this magical machine—the human body, the moving temple of God or the chariot for the soul. Mother Prakriti has exhibited her marvellous skill and maximum dexterity in constructing this marvellous machine. If you seriously ponder over for a while over the structure and working of this wonderful machine that is our body you will be struck with awe and wonder.

The cells of these glands are endowed with marvellous intelligence. There are many endocrine glands and they all work in perfect unison and harmony with each other and thus the normal functioning of the body is maintained. If the function of one gland is disturbed a vicious circle will be formed. These internal secretory glands pour directly into the blood stream, their secretions in such quantities as are necessary to keep up a balance of bodily activity.

The various ductless glands of the body are the pineal, the pituitary, the thyroid, the parathyroid, the thymus, the adrenals or the supra-renals, the gonads or the generative glands, and the islets of Langerhans. Chemists are now manufacturing some of these glandular products artificially from lower animals. Doctors administer these extracts or solutions to patients either by means of injections or by mouth to replace the secretions of the patients' glands when they are not functioning properly. Pituitrin, the active principle of the pituitary gland, pancreatic extract, known as insulin, for the treatment of diabetes, adrenalin, the active principle of the adrenal glands, thyroxin, the active principle of the thyroid gland, and Para-thormone from the parathyroid have been prepared by the chemists.

The pineal gland or pineal body is of the size of a pea, and has the shape of a cone. It is imbedded in the brain above the top of the spinal column near the middle of the skull.

It contains some gritty calcareous particles called brain sand. It is the receiving instrument of the wireless telegraphy of the mind. It receives the thought messages from distant telepathists. Some regard the pineal gland as the seat of the soul. It functions most vigorously in the practice of telepathy, and plays a tremendous part in thought-transference. Occultists consider this as the sixth sense.

The pituitary gland is located at the base of the brain and produces several kinds of hormones. It has got two lobes, viz., the anterior lobe and the posterior lobe. This gland has much to do with the development of our height, weight and general contour, the character of the hair, the texture of the skin and the cast of features. This is a small body weighing six grams. Research workers are not in agreement regarding the number of hormones produced by the anterior lobe of the pituitary, but in general four are recognised, viz., the growth, gonadotropic, lactogenic, threotropic principles. The anterior lobe of the pituitary body promotes skeletal growth. Hyper-activity of the anterior lobe is a cause for premature sex-development. The important functions of the posterior lobe are stimulation of the non-striated muscle fibres and control of the carbohydrate metabolism. Any deficiency in the secretion of the posterior lobe causes muscular weakness and a slowing up of carbohydrate metabolism with greatly increased sugar tolerance. Excessive functioning of this gland causes gigantism or unusually large hands, feet or nose, aggressiveness and persistence. Any deficiency produces a normally intelligent, obedient, good-natured and fickle-minded man. It also leads to dwarfism, excessive obesity and retardation of sexual development.

The pituitary gland functions more vigorously after the removal of the thyroid. But it does not take over all the duties of the thyroid. If the function of the pituitary gland is impaired or lost, the thyroid gland begins to function more vigorously. This is a balancing action on nature's part. Similarly when the kidneys are in a diseased condition the skin works more vigorously and *vice versa*. In summer the skin functions more energetically and so we perspire more profusely. In winter the activity of the kidneys is accelerated and we pass more urine. Micturition is more frequent also. This sort of balancing work in the harmony of nature is done by the intelligent Prakriti under the direct guidance of the Lord of all nature. The Sattwa Guna of the Prakriti is characterised by intelligence.

The thyroid gland consists of two lobes which are attached to the sides of the lower portion of the larynx. In a normal individual it weighs from 20 to 25 grams. The secretion of this gland plays a very vital part in keeping up a proper balance over nutritional and growth process in human beings. The active principle of the secretions of this gland is called thyroxin. The general effect of the thyroid hormone on metabolism is a regulation of the rate of oxidation in the body. A lack of thyroid secretion results in dwarfism, deficient muscular activity, lower bodily temperature, slower breathing rate, a depressed activity and underdeveloped and functionally deficient sex-glands. Goitre is a morbid enlargement of the thyroid gland. This is due to complete absence or marked deficiency of the iodine necessary for the normal functioning of the gland. Regular consumption of foods rich in iodine will help in preventing goitre. Children who suffer from cretinism show considerable improvement if they take thyroxin. Excessive functioning of the thyroid induces rapid physical development and sex-changes, increased restlessness and irritability.

The para-thyroids are closely attached to the thyroids. They are four in number. They weigh in all not more than two grains. The secretion from the para-thyroid controls the calcium content of the blood. The proper functioning of the glands is of paramount importance. Calcium helps the clotting of blood, and the muscular tone and the formation of the skeleton. An insufficiency of calcium in the blood is shown by the appearance of certain diseases. Complete removal of these glands results in a condition known as tetany which is characterised by painful spasmodic contractions of the muscles of the extremities, i.e., hands and legs. The calcium content of the blood is considerably diminished. The heart, lungs and the temperature of the body are also affected. The patient dies if proper treatment is not given. Administration of an extract of parathyroid promptly restores the sufferer to a normal condition.

The thymus is situated in the upper region of the chest along the trachea or wind-pipe. Removal of the thymus in human beings induces disordered development of the skeleton and results in defects like ricket, etc. The thymus is particularly important in childhood as it helps the physical and mental development. Early decline of thymic activity results in sexual precocity, whereas persistent thymus activity causes delayed puberty.

The adrenal glands are of yellow colour. They are two in number. Each weighs about four grams. Each is situated above the kidney. They produce two major hormones, viz., adrenalin and cortin. The secretion from the medullary portion of the adrenal gland is called adrenalin. This is widely used as a drug. It stops bleeding by inducing contraction of the arteries and capillaries and maintains muscular tone. A deficiency of adrenalin causes lowered blood pressure, lack of muscular tone and loss of strength. The secretions of the cortex control sexual maturity. Over-activity of the cortex portion of the adrenal causes masculine traits in women, such as the growth of a beard, harsh voice, etc. Hypertrophy of the cortex causes precocious sexual development. Morbid affection of the cortical portion causes Addison's disease. When cortical extract is injected, the patient shows signs of improvement. The adrenal glands assist in sexual development especially in early life, maintain muscular tone, including arterial tension and exert a protective influence against bacterial infection.

The generative glands (Gonads) produce internal secretions which affect the individual both mentally and physically. The gonads exercise deep psychological and physiological influence on men. These secretions determine the proper development of the specific male and female characteristics, such as voice, hairy condition, bodily outline, size, etc.

The pancreas is a gland that secretes a digestive juice called pancreatic juice which is poured through the pancreatic duct into the small intestines. In the midst of the lobules which secrete the pancreatic juice there are small tissues known as the islets of Langerhans. These tissues secrete a substance called insulin which is directly absorbed in the blood. This hormone plays a very important part in the metabolism of carbohydrates. If there is any deficiency of this hormone insulin through disease of the islets of Langerhans, diabetes-mellitus is produced. The chief symptom of diabetes is increase of sugar in the urine. Doctors inject now an extract known as Insulin prepared from the pancreas of healthy animals for the treatment of diabetes-mellitus.

A hormone does not influence directly the endocrine gland from which it originates. On the contrary the active principles secreted by a gland may strikingly influence certain other endocrine glands. For instance, the ovarian follicular hormone does not affect the ovary directly, but exerts its effect upon the secondary sex organs. The ovarian hormone exerts a restraining effect on the anterior pituitary.

The internal secretions or hormones play a very important role in influencing the structure of our body, health, complexion, personality. Each endocrine gland must play its part in perfect tune and harmony with its companion. Then only will there be physiological harmony. Then only will the internal administration or government within the body run smoothly. Then only will you enjoy perfect health and peace.

CHAPTER II

Health and Hygiene

1. BATH

Cleanliness is next to Godliness. A bath daily in cold water in the early mornings before sunrise is really bracing, invigorating, energising and refreshing. The best time for a bath is early morning before sunrise, because the water that gets cooled during the night evolves much oxygen at this time. The sick and the convalescents, the old and people of delicate health may take a warm water bath. The application of soap in a tropical climate is injurious. It keeps the skin dry. Nature supplies a little oil to the body for keeping it smooth and soft through the secretion of the sebaceous glands of the skin. Ignorant fashionable man removes this natural secretion by application of soap and wastes his money. If soaps are not manufactured properly they corrode the skin. Rub the body vigorously with a rough towel. This will open all the pores of the skin and cleanse the latter properly. Resort always to easy natural methods that cost nothing. If you like, you can use a mixture of soap-nut powder and green-gram powder for cleasing the skin. This is cheap and very cooling also.

A plunge bath in the running water of rivers is very exhilarating and strengthening. A shower bath is also very enjoyable. Baths in sulphur springs cure diseases of the skin. Louis Kuhne's system of baths is highly beneficial. A cold hip bath prevents wet-dreams. A tepid hip bath stops renal colic and helps the free flow of menstrual fluid and urine. A steam bath is useful in rheumatism. Tepid sponging is useful in fevers for bringing down the temperature.

Do not take a cold bath immediately after performing Asans or any kind of exercises. Allow the body to cool down first. Wait for an hour. Never bathe soon after your meals as it will interfere with your digestion.

2. THE BENEFITS OF A SUN-BATH

Sun is the source of all energy and power. You derive energy and power from the sun. If the sun does not shine for a day or two on account of clouds your vitality falls to a low level and you are not in good spirits. Flowers, plants, animals and men rejoice as soon as the sun rises above the horizon. The sun supplies energy to all plants and living beings and yet its energy is never exhausted. Its energy is inexhaustible because it derives its energy from the inexhaustible source—Atma, the "Sun of suns."

The rays of the sun bestow on us wonderful health. The Rig Vedas have glorified the rising sun. The Ayurvedas have extolled its efficacy. The Rishis have sung its praise in a variety of ways. The Tantras sing its glory in the Mantra: "*Japakusum Sankasham*—the rising sun is as red as the Japa flower."

Build your house on the western bank of a river, lake or tank. Then you will daily enjoy the reflected light which is more beneficial and potent than the direct rays. The rays of the rising sun are blessings from God for the preservation of health as well as for the cure of diseases. The rays of the sun possess antiseptic and germicidal properties. Expose your blankets, bedsheets, pillows and mattresses to the sun once in every fifteen days. In the rays of the sun you will find a cheap and and easily available tonic, a disinfectant, an antiseptic and a potent germicide.

Sunlight as a healer of leprosy and various other skin diseases was known to the ancients. The latter built temples dedicated to the Sun. The temple of Konarak was built upon a tradition that Samba, the son of Sri Krishna, was stricken with leprosy because he saw his father in the act of connubial pleasure. When entreated to be forgiven Krishna asked Samba to worship the Sun in order to be freed of the loathsome disease. Accordingly he did so and was cured. In Egypt the Sun God is Ra; in Greece, Apollo;

in Phoenicia the Sun; and in Syria also the sun and the moon were worshipped. In France and Germany the peasants even now take off their hats to the rays of the sun. In India the Martanda Mandir in Kashmir; the sun-temple at Vikrampur; the Suryakund of Benares are further examples of the deities of sunworship. There is a Vrita called Surya-Vrita when people do not eat fish and take simple and unsalted food. The sun is worshipped and looked at by the Hindus when they take bath in the morning with the sloka: "*Japakusum Sankasham,*" etc.

There is a system of physical exercise called Suryanamaskar and the Raja Saheb of Aundh is a great propounder of it. The Prince of Aundh, like his father, is a great votary of Suryanamaskar. Recently at the request of the students at Bangalore he demonstrated the Suryanamaskar in many colleges there and explained its benefits. Do Suryanamaskar in the early morning. The morning sun gives out ultra-violet rays as does also the evening sun. If persons suffering from leprosy and other skin diseases strip themselves off all clothing and remain naked in the sun till their body is properly tanned, then the sun rays will penetrate their body and work wonders there. Only the head must be protected from the sun. Besides leprosy, tuberculosis, rheumatism, obesity, anaemia, neurasthenia, eczema, colds, coughs, rickets, diseases of the teeth, etc., can also be treated with sun rays.

Wear a thin light garment and walk on the western bank of a river, on the west side of the sea, a lake or a tank early morning at sunrise. Run also. You will doubtless enjoy a sun-bath. Practise Asans and physical exercises. Expose your mouth to the rays of the rising sun. Open it wide. Let the rays penerate your nostrils also. Close your eyes when you expose your mouth. Let the sun's rays fall on the closed eyes for two or three minutes. This will improve your short sight. Practise deep-breathing exercises and Pranayam. The various parts of the body should receive a regulated sun-bath. Turn the body round frequently.

Bask in the sun. Expose your body to the rays of the sun for a short time. Lie down on the ground on a blanket or lie on a cot. Expose your back to the rays of the sun. If the rays are very hot cover your back with a green plantain leaf. Remain thus for fifteen or thirty minutes till you perspire freely. This will prove useful in lumbago and rheumatism and diseases of the skin.

The Rishis and sages of yore who had knowledge of the curative power of the rays of the sun revealed the mysteries of the sun and its beneficial rays and the uses of this radiant energy. But you don't care to read and learn them. You want to borrow everything from the West. What a sad lamentable state! Study Aditya Hridaya daily. Perform Suryanamaskar daily. Give Arghya to the sun at the times of Sandhya. You will then have wonderful health and vigour and vitality. Even in the West doctors are using the rays of the sun as a powerful therapeutic agent in the treatment of diseases. They call this helio-therapy. In sanatoriums on the Alps the consumptive patients are directly exposed to the mild rays of the sun. In olden days in India babies with bare bodies were put in the cradle and exposed to the rising sun. In California boys and girls now take sunbaths. They swing in the open air with bare bodies in specially constructed swings.

Whence comes the mysterious power in the sun which causes the seeds to germinate and the flowers to turn into fruits? Whence comes this radiant energy in the sun which bestows wonderful health, power and vigour to living beings? Whence in the sun comes this power to heal? Whence comes in the sun the vital energy that invigorates and galvanises the young and rejuvenates and vitalises the old? Whence comes in the sun this vegetative vigour which enables the plants to synthetise the vitamins? The sun derives its power and energy from Atma or the Eternal or the Absolute, the Sun of suns, the Light of lights, the source of everything, the first cause of all causes, the storehouse of all energies. Brahman willed. The sun came into being to bestow health and happiness to all beings. Repeat the twelve names of the Sun at sunrise : "Mitrayai Namah; Ravaye Namah; Suryayah Namah; Bhanuvai Namah; Savitraye Namah; Adityayi Namah; Bhaskaraya Namah."

He who repeats this at sunrise early in the morning will possess wonderful health, vigour and vitality. He will be free from any kind of the diseases of the eye. He will have powerful eyesight. Pray to the sun in the early morning before sunrise: "O Lord, Suryanarayan, the Eye of the World, the Eye of the Virat Purusha, give me health and strength, vigour and vitality." Offer arghya to the sun in the three Sandhyas (morning, noon and sunset).

Repeat the prayer of the Isavasya Upanishad, sloka 15 and 16: "The face of Truth is covered by a golden vessel. Remove, O Sun, the covering, for the law of Truth, that I may behold it." "O Pooshan (Sun Nourisher), the only seer (whole traveller of the heavens), controller of all (Yama), Surya, son of Prajapati, disperse thy rays and gather up thy burning light; I behold thy glorious form, I am He, the Purusha within Thee." In the words of Yajur Veda, "O Sun of suns! You are all-energy, give me energy; you are all-strength, give me strength; you are all-powerful, give me power."

I always prostrate before the Sun God, the beautiful Lord of the world, the immortal, the quintessence of Vedanta, the auspicious, the absolute knowledge, the all-full Brahman, Lord of the Devas, ever pure, the one true consciousness of the world, the Lord of Gods and men, the preceptor of Devas, the crest jewel of the three worlds (Bhu, Bhuva and Svah), the form of the heart of Vishnu, Brahman, and Siva, the dispeller of darkness and the giver of light.

3. SLEEP

Man works hard in daytime so that he may get what he deserves most. He is tossed about hither and thither by the two currents Raga-Dwesha. So he gets tired. Nature takes him to her bosom at night to soothe his tired nerves and brain, to refresh him, and to supply him with fresh energy and vigour so that he may continue his activities the next day. She makes him go to sleep. Sleep is a physiological phenomenon by which the mind, the brain and all the organs get rest for some hours. During sleep the mind goes back to its source. There is manolaya or temporary absorption of the mind into its cause—the Avidya.

Vedantins make a deep study of sleep and draw conclusions about the all-blissful Atma, the silent witness of the state of deep sleep. The mind assumes a seed-like state in deep sleep. The samskaras and vasanas become latent. All vritties subside. The mind that was working in the brain during the waking state moves through Sushumna Nadi into the heart and it rests on Atma. The Chaitanya or intelligence that is associated with the deep sleep state is Prajna. Karana Sarira or seed body or Anandamaya Kosha or blissful sheath operates during deep sleep. The Jiva is very near to Atma. A thin veil of ignorance separates him from Atma, just as the thin veil separates the husband from his wife. The husband rejoices as soon as his wife removes the veil. Even so the individual soul rejoices as soon as the veil of ignorance is removed and when he comes face to face with Brahman. Mind, Prana, Indriyas and the body derive their power from the one silent witness of all minds. It is the soul that really moves the indriyas, mind and body and Prakriti works. So Atma is Sarva Karta (all-doer) and also Akarta (non-doer), Sarva Bhokta (all-enjoyer) and also Abhokta (non-enjoyer).

Sleep is nature's tonic for a healthy life. The more sound sleep one has, the more healthy he would be. The hours of sleep necessary depend on your physical and mental capacity for resisting fatigue. Without a sufficiency of sleep, you will have no efficiency. The amount of sleep required varies with age, temperament and amount of work done. According to an old adage : "There should be six hours of sleep for a man, seven for a woman and eight for a fool." As age advances people require less sleep. Ten hours' sleep is necessary for a child. In old men above 60 years, six hours of sleep may be sufficient. Adults who work hard may sleep for eight hours. Medical men and psychologists are paying great attention these days to the question of sleep.

Sleep for six hours is quite sufficient for every individual. Go to bed at 10 o'clock and get up at 4 a.m. An old adage says : "Early to bed, early to rise makes a man healthy, wealthy and wise." Napoleon Bonaparte believed in only four hours' sleep. Too much sleep makes a man dull and lethargic. What is required is quality of sleep. Even if you have a sound dreamless sleep for 1 or 2 hours, you will be perfectly refreshed. There is no benefit to be derived from rolling in the bed for hours together. Too much sleep causes premature decay and weakens brain power.

Avoid going late to bed. When you sleep keep all the windows and doors of your bed-room well open. The more oxygen you inhale during your sleep, the more refreshed you will feel throughout the next day. Do not take drugs to get sleep. If you cannot sleep naturally take a brisk walk in the open air for fifteen minutes and then go to bed. You are sure to have refreshing sleep.

Digestion takes place at night. Consequently you should take a light meal at night. Strong coffee or tea should not be taken at night. Sleep on the sides, especially on the right side. This helps to empty the stomach and allow the Surya Nadi or Pingala to flow. Food will be digested easily if the Solar Nadi flows at night. Keep the same time daily for sleep. Wear loose clothing. Do not cover yourself with heavy blankets or clothings.

Relax the body and mind when you go to sleep. Repeat some prayer or sublime slokas of Gita or Upanishads before you go to bed. Roll the beads for ten minutes and meditate on the form of the Lord and Divine attributes. Do not build castles in the air. Give up scheming and planning now. If you have ill-feeling against any one, forget it. Have pleasant thoughts only.

Keeping wide awake throughout night is called vigil. You will derive incalculable benefits if you practise vigil on Vaikunta Ekadashi, Sivaratri and Gokulashtami, the birthday of Lord Krishna. You can practise vigil on every Ekadashi also. Complete fasting helps in the control of sleep. Control of sleep by taking recourse to tea is not desirable. You will not gain spiritual strength thus as you have to depend upon an extraneous drug.

Half of your lifetime is wasted in sleep. Those spiritual aspirants who want to do rigorous sadhan should reduce their period of sleep gradually. They can get real rest from meditation. For three months reduce the sleeping period by half an hour. Go to bed at 10-30 and get up at 4 a.m. During the next three months go to bed at 11 p.m. and get up at 4 a.m. Four hours' sleep will amply suffice. You should not sleep in the daytime. In course of time you should not become Gudakesa (conqueror of sleep), like Arjun and Lakshman, and rest in that all-blissful, sleepless sleep, the Nirvikalpa Samadhi of Yogins.

4. YOGIC DIET

A Yogic diet is that which helps the aspirant to keep the mind calm and to curb the restless indriyas. A Yogic diet helps him to squeeze out the rajas from his mind and fill the mind with sattwa and to practise unceasing meditation. All the indriyas should be filled with pure materials. Then only the mind will attain one-pointedness. Then only it will become pure. Then only you can attain self-realisation. The eyes should see the picture of your Ishtam or any other holy object. The ears should hear the Upanishads, Ramayana or Bhagwat. The tongue should speak of matters that concern God. These are all pure materials or food for the indriyas.

The right kind of food is most important. Half the illnesses of the nation are due to an ill-balanced diet. There is no mystery about diet. It can be learnt very easily. A correct diet is a fundamental factor in the maintenance of perfect health and a high standard of vitality. Good food is not expensive. A well-balanced diet is not costly. It is knowledge of dietetics that we hopelessly lack. The Ministers of Health should tackle this problem of diet for the young, adults and the convalescents. The Board of Education should train experts in dietetics.

Unwholesome stale food or any kind of unsuitable diet or drink produces irritating poisons in the blood which causes various kinds of disorders. The liver and the kidneys are taxed by high or luxurious living. Rich people who lead a life of dissipation suffer from organic diseases of the liver and the kidneys. They have to pay a heavy penalty, because they have violated the laws of nature and the rules of health.

Drinking alcohol affects the liver. Eating meat, beaf, etc., affects the kidneys. Nature puts a check on the man who violates her laws by inducing chronic structural diseases of vital organs. If you take too much of sugar or sweetmeats, you may suffer from diabetes and you are forced by nature to give up sugar. This is the punishment by Mother Prakriti on her impertinent children who transgress her laws. As all palatable food is tempting man takes more food than is actually necessary for the upkeep of the body. He eats three times as much as is necessary to keep him well. He unduly overloads his stomach. He loses control over the tongue and the power of discrimination when he sits in front of the tempting dishes. He says: "I must eat to my heart's content today. It does not matter even if I load my stomach and suffer from dyspepsia. I will take a strong purgative and a dose of some carminative mixture in the morning." Mark here ! How powerful is the tongue ! How powerful is Maya !

The nature of food that is taken determines the character of individuals. Carnivorous food makes men callous and bestial. It excites the passion and renders the intellect gross. A meat-eater cannot become a philosopher and a sage. His intellect is so dull that he cannot solve the problems of life herein and hereafter. The intellect is rendered keen, subtle and sharp by a vegetable diet. A vegetable diet is highly conducive to sublime thinking and divine contemplation. It gives greater vitality than animal foods. Beans, tomatoes, potatoes, raddish, carrot, ladies fingers, cucumbers, drumsticks, spinach, green leafy vegetables are all pure, delicious and nutritious food and can be taken with much advantage.

The diet should be carefully well-chosen and arranged. Condiments, tea, coffee, alcohol, foods that are rich in starch, sugars and fats, and all stimulating drinks should be avoided. Fresh fruits, salads and raw vegetables, cheese, nuts, cereals, wholemeal bread, soya beans, dried fruits, cream, milk, barley, honey, dates, almonds are highly beneficial. Raw foods make better blood and build better bodies and should therefore make up at least eighty per cent of the diet. Live on juicy fruits for a week. This will help greatly towards the elimination of impurities from the system. Raw foods are better than cooked ones. The former are more vitalising than the latter.

Indigestion or dyspepsia induced by an unnaturally heavy meal or unwholesome irritating food or unsuitable diet will cause all kinds of reflex effects on the nerve centres. Masticate the food slowly. Eat only when you are hungry. Eat slowly. Drink plenty of water after finishing the food. Do not drink water between meals as it will dilute the gastric juice and will cause indigestion and other stomach complaints.

The mouth is the gate-keeper of the digestive system. It should always be kept sweet and clean by rinsing the mouth with a solution of potassium permanganate several times soon after taking food. If the mouth is kept unclean, if the food particles are allowed to stick in the crevices of the teeth, pyorrhoea with its concomitant complications will result. Many germs breed in an unclean mouth. Cleansing of the teeth is of paramount importance. Chewing of a few neem leaves keeps the mouth sweet and clean. Neem leaves act as a powerful germicide. Cleanse the teeth with mustard oil and salt. This is a very useful combination.

We require a variety of foods with a variety of contents and properties. Variety in food is necessary but too many different kinds at one time are not good. The fewer the kinds the better. Mother Prakriti provides judiciously and amply all our needs and varies the contents of foods in accordance with our needs.

A simple diet, containing a mimimum of unnecessary food or waste, will throw less strain upon the kidneys than a rich diet will do. Proper diet ensures healthy and supple tissues by preventing the accumulation of waste in the system. An eminent doctor says: "The perfect food consists of honey, cream, hot water, oat-meal, lemon-juice, grated apple and ground hazel-nuts which contain all the vitamins."

(a) Honey: A Food and Tonic

Honey is a food and a tonic. Honey is a first class food. It is very easily digestible. It is assimilated quite readily also. This is a most nutritious natural food. It will strengthen a weak heart, a weak brain and a weak stomach.

Honey is a product of the nectar of flowers. It is a mistake to say that honey is gathered by bees from flowers. Bees are nature's Halwais. They manufacture sweets better, finer and healthier than any sweetmeat maker with all his skill, dexterity, ingenuity and many ingredients can ever make.

Green plants manufacture sugar for their own use. This is carried with the cell sap to the different parts of the plant either for direct assimilation or future use. All the flowering plants concentrate a quick supply of food at the base or at the bottom part of their flowers to help the proper growth of the ovaries. The excess solution is thrown out at the base of the flowers. This thrown out solution of the cell sap with sugar is known as 'nectar.' This nectar is changed into honey in their mouths by the honey-bees. Every hive imparts a new flavour because in every hive the nectar is drawn from different flowers and plants.

Honey contains all the mineral elements found in the human body. It contains 80% of nutriment in the most assimilable form. It contains the sugars levulose and dextrose, formic acid, iron and various accessory components. It contains enzymes. These enzymes disintegrate or break up complex foods into substances that can be easily digested and absorbed. Honey does not require digestion at all. It is ready for absorption into the blood without any change. It goes into the blood stream directly. It should form an article of your diet. A teaspoonful of honey will keep the stomach in order for ever.

Honey is a heart stimulant. It is useful in cases of malnutrition. It should be given for general physical repair. Honey kills bacteria and thus enables the body to overcome diseases. Disease germs cannot grow in honey. Honey is substituted for orange juice and cod-liver oil. It is useful in bronchial catarrh, sore throat, coughs and colds. Diabetic patients can take honey with advantage.

Honey also acts as a laxative. It enters into the combination of Chavan Prash and other kalpas. It is taken in combination with amalaka fruits as a kalpa. As soon as a child is born its tongue is smeared with honey. This is the first food that the child takes.

Honey can be taken with milk, cream or butter. It is a restorative after serious illness. It invigorates, energises and vitalises the system. It improves health. It is more stimulating than alcohol and helps weak digestion.

Honey is a diffusible stimulant. If you take a tablespoonful of honey in hot water when you are tired or exhausted by over-exertion, it will brace you up immediately. You will become strong and active again. If the honey is bitter do not take it. Soak 10 almonds in water at night. Remove the skin in the morning. Take them in the morning with one or two tablespoonfuls of honey. This is a potent brain tonic.

(b) Milk and Its Products

Milk is an ideal diet. It is a perfect and complete food in itself. It contains all the nutritive principles in a well-balanced proportion. You can live on milk alone. In India there is a sect among the sadhus known as 'Dudhadharis.' They take no other food but milk and yet they possess sound and perfect health. One man has lived on a strictly milk diet for more than fifty years. He has never been ill even for a day during that period. He is healthy and well-nourished. Charaka Rishi says: "Give no other medicine to your patients but milk and cure them one and all." Milk contains proteins (casein), fat, milk, sugar and mineral salts. All infants grow properly on an exclusive milk diet. The sick recover their health and strength when put on milk alone. Take plenty of milk. Not only is it rich in proteins and minerals, but it also contains the four most important vitamins.

Curd, lassey, cheese, whey, butter, cream, ghee, etc., are the products of milk. Lassey can be made out of milk or curd. Equal parts of milk and water with sugar or one part of curd with four parts of water and some sugar forms lassey.

Lassey is very cooling. It is taken in the morning. It opens the bowels. It is useful in consumption. It kills the T.B. germs. This is taken by the Punjabis and the people of Hindustan and Bengal.

The clear liquid left after curd or cheese has been separated is called whey. This is highly beneficial in constipation and diseases of the stomach and intestines. It is a very good food for invalids and convalescents. It is also easily digestible.

Buttermilk is very cooling to the system. It quenches thirst. It is useful in diseases of the stomach and intestines. It is useful in dysentery. The lactic acid contained in buttermilk kills the pathogenetic germs that may be present in the stomach and bowels.

Fruits and milk form a very healthy, wholesome diet. This diet helps the concentration of mind. It is the diet of Rishis and Raja Yogins. This is also the diet of Hatha Yogins who practise Pranayam vigorously. Try to live on milk and fruits on Sundays and Ekadashis. The value of milk as a tissue-building agent when taken alone or in combination with fresh fruits cannot be too strongly emphasised. Milk is a perfect diet containing as it does all the dietetic principles in a well-balanced proportion.

(c) Fruits and Health

Among the different foods, fruits stand foremost in importance in the Yogi's menu or regimen. The curative effects of fresh juicy fruits are astonishing. These juices cleanse the tissues and throw out the morbid materials from the bodily system. They fill the body with vitalising or life-giving mineral salts, potassium, sodium, manganese, iron, calcium, etc. Dr. J. H. Kellogg says: "Fruit juices contain vitamins and food minerals especially iron and lime, which are indispensable in many body processes and which need to be given in great abundance under the conditions present in disease. When the body is struggling under conditions which cripple its functions such as overworked liver or kidneys especially, a large intake of vitamins in the form of grape juice or other fruit juices will invigorate the curative forces of the body and produce effects which are unapproachable by even the most powerful drugs."

Tomatoes contain citric acid and mallic acid and a small quantity of oxalic acid. It contains large quantities of five of the six vitamins. Cooking partially destroys the vitamin content. Therefore tomatoes should be eaten raw. Tomatoes contain the salt potash, lime, magnesia and iron. They exercise a beneficial effect on the liver, kidneys and other organs. They also cure constipation.

The orange is a blood-purifier. It tones up the entire system of the body. It invigorates and energises. It is a good appetiser. It is very rich in vitamin C. It also contains vitamin B and vitamin A. (Vitamins are the essentials of man's existence.) It possesses anti-scorbutic properties and hence cures scurvy. It cures constipation also. It promotes growth and prevents rickets. When in season it should form a regular part of your diet. It supplies nutrition to the body in a small bulk. It helps concentration and meditation. It is a sattwic article of diet. Live on orange juice for a week or fortnight and practise vigorous meditation. Orange juice mixed with fresh grape juice makes a very good tonic. This is very useful in anaemia or poverty of blood, general debility, rickets, etc.

Banana or plantain fruit contains A, B, C and D vitamins. This is a very good soothing food. You can live on milk and bananas alone. They are very nutritious. They promote growth, augment vigour and add flesh to the body. The fully ripe fruits act as a laxative. Take one or two fruits at bed time. You will have free movement of the bowels in the morning.

Mangoes contain sugar and highly refined turpentine in them. They also contain iron and other useful acids. They are useful in rheumatism, diarrhoea, diabetes. Mangoes and milk is a wonderful combination. You can live on this diet for two or three months.

Pomegranates are also very invigorating, cooling and strengthening. The juice is very refreshing and toning.

Those who want to supply energy to their system quickly should take this juice. Those who deliver fiery lectures on the platform will derive immense benefit by taking this juice. They will be supplied with fresh energy and will be quite fit for the next lecture in a short space of time.

The pineapple is an old fashioned domestic remedy for quinsy and ordinary throat affections of an acute nature. A pineapple is very beneficial in case of enlargement of spleen. Take one fruit daily. Papaya contains the active principle of alkaloid papain. The latter digests food readily. Papaya fruits should not be ignored from the daily diet. Bael fruit also is very cooling. A sherbet can be formed out of this fruit and drunk in summer. It is useful in dysentery. It stops the passing of blood and heals the ulcers that may have formed in the lower bowels.

Jambul fruits are useful in diabetes-mellitus. They remove the excess of sugar in the urine. An apple is a very nutritious fruit. The proverb is: "An apple a day keeps the doctor away." Apple and cream is a very good combination in cases of high blood pressure. The chikku or sapota is a blood purifier. It enriches the blood quantitatively and qualitatively. It contains iron in abundance.

The all-fruit diet is the finest eliminating medium. In the treatment of lumbago the patient is put on a diet of oranges alone. The uric acid that is accumulated in the system is eliminated quickly by this diet. The body becomes light when one lives on fruits alone. Tamas is destroyed. You can conquer sleep if you live on a fruit diet alone. Those who live on fruits alone experience a peculiar, inexpressible ananda or bliss. They sometimes feel that they have no body. Some people who live on fruits feel weakness in the beginning, because their stomachs were habituated to heavy starchy food.. They used to load their stomachs to the brim. After sometime through force of the new habit the feeling of weakness will vanish. The all-fruit diet can be carried on for two weeks or more with ease by most people. When all other remedies fail in the treatment of chronic diseases, an all-fruit diet may work wonders.

Friends ! Why do you take carnivorous foods and spoil your health ? Carnivorous foods excite passion and make the mind restless. Fruits exercise a soothing influence on the mind and subdue passion. Man leads an artificial life in these days of modern civilization and scientific advancement. He lives on patent foods, drinks alcohol, puts on tight collars, attends theatres, eats all sorts of things in hotels and restaurants, forgets God and the goal of life, leads an unnatural life of dissipation and meets with various sorts of diseases and premature death. What a sad, lamentable state !

If you take pure food you will have a pure mind. Mind is formed out of the subtlest essence of food. If you have purity of mind, you will remember God or Atma. If you always remember Atma, the knots of the heart, viz., Avidya, Kama, Karma (ignorance, desire and action) will be rent asunder. You will attain Moksha.

If you would attain longevity and possess good health and vigour you must go back to nature. Lead a simple natural life with high sublime thinking. Live on fruits. Develop ethical virtues, control the indriyas and mind, practise meditation, realise the Self and be for ever free.

5. FASTING

Fasting is a form of tapas to destroy the effects of evil samskaras and purify oneself quickly. It is a kind of prayaschitta to nullify the effects of evil actions. It is a sort of self-punishment. Fasting is a sacred vrita amongst the Hindus. They take a complete fast on Sivaratri and Gokulasthami days. They do not take even a drop of water during these days. Some religious-minded persons fast on every Ekadashi day. Fasting subdues passion. Even Christians observe Lent, for 40 days (from Ash Wednesday to Easter Eve) are devoted to fasting and penitence in commemoration of the fast of their Saviour in the wilderness. Mohamedans fast during Ramzan. Fasting helps in controlling the mind and makes the mind sattwic. Manu has prescribed Krishcharata Vrita and Chandrayana Vrita for purification of mind and destroying the evil effects of great offences.

Fasting has in numberless cases restored health when everything else had failed. If you fast as soon as a disease is manifested, it will soon disappear and many serious complications will be avoided. If you feel feverish, if you suffer from dyspepsia fast for a day and you will be cured immediately. Nowadays many have recognised and realised the value of fasting. They resort to fasting whenever any form of ill-health manifests itself and save big doctor's bills. Medicine only helps nature. A doctor may ruin the health of a patient by his injudicious treatment. Nature is your reliable guide, doctor, friend and nurse. Seek her help always. She is ever ready to serve you with warm affection. Charaka Rishi recommends fasting for the cure of many chronic diseases. Fasting is nature's greatest curative agent. The fast gives an opportunity to nature to cleanse the system and remove the materials that clog certain organs or parts. It is a very efficacious therapeutic agent. Many kinds of poisonous materials and toxins are eliminated by fasting. Fasting reduces fat.

Fasting does not impair vitality. It does not produce weakness and loss of weight. Some people are unnecessarily alarmed when they hear the word 'fasting.' Strength and vitality are usually increased by fasting. The mind becomes clear during fasting. The body becomes very light.

The practice of fasting may be disgusting in the beginning for some persons. But later on they themselves will take great delight in it. You will be troubled by hunger on the first day and on the second day. From the third day you will have no difficulty. You will have no appetite. Do not allow the mind to think of various articles of diet during fasting. Practise rigorous meditation during this period. The indriyas are calm now. You can do much meditation. Practise fasting for a day to start with and through force of habit you can gradually increase the period to a week. When you break the fast take some fruit juice, preferably orange juice. Do not load the stomach with solid food all at once. Gluttons are unfit for long fasts. If the mind does a wrong action, if it hurts others' feelings seriously punish it by observing a fast. It will come under your control gradually.

If you find it difficult to observe complete fast even for a day at least observe partial fast. Do not take anything in the daytime. Take milk and fruits at night. Or take fruit-juice only. Do not take any solid food but take only fruit-juice. Continue the fruit-juice fast for two or three days.

You should drink water copiously when you observe fast for 4 or 5 days to flush out the system. What do the municipal people do when the sewers are clogged? Do they not flush it with plenty of water? You should do the same thing when your system is clogged. The water drunk may be flavoured slightly with a little of the juice of an orange, a lemon or grapes. Take an enema of soap water in the early morning to cleanse the bowels thoroughly. Just as a car after thorough overhauling looks like a new car and runs smoothly, so also our body which is clogged by over-eating and stuffing of all sorts of food, gets thoroughly overhauled by fasting and becomes like a new machine and works very efficiently.

Fasting develops will-power. Mahatma Gandhiji had developed his will-power considerably through fasting. He was a great votary of fasting. If anything went wrong in the Ashram, if any one conducted himself in a wrong manner, he would fast for some days. He took the burden and sins of others on himself by fasting. He fasted for effecting Hindu-Muslim unity. He had a long fast of 45 days for the political and economical good or freedom of the country.

Fasting is the message of the heart. By fasting you can melt the heart of even a hard-hearted man. By fasting you can influence anybody. By fasting you can make the Indra and other Devatas to serve you. Fasting has magical influence indeed.

Fast and calm your emotions and passion. Fast and be healthy. Fast and control the tongue and other indriyas. Fast and destroy your sins. Fast and eliminate the poison from your system. Fast and control sleep. Fast and pray.

Fast, purify and meditate, realise the self and be free. Fast and shine with divine splendour and glory.

6. DISEASES

(*Adi-Vyadi*)

All chronic, long-standing and functional derangements or ailments are invariably associated with definite abnormal conditions in the mechanism, tissues and organs of the body. Disease is only being *dis* and *ease*, i.e., not at ease. It is the result of a violation of some laws of nature. Nature wants every one to be healthy and strong. If you are weak it indicates that your organs or the various cells of your body are not functioning properly. Remove the cause of the disease. Do not play with the symptoms of disease. It is much more simple to prevent than cure.

You must treat the cause of any disease. This is the rational method of treatment of any disease or impaired health. There is no use in suppressing the symptoms. If the root-cause is not eradicated, and if the symptoms are suppressed for the time-being, the disease will assume an aggravated chronic form. The only rational method of treatment is that which takes into consideration the causes and directs all its efforts towards the restoration of normal functions throughout the system.

Nature does everything. Medicines help nature in the recuperative work and the regenerative or constructive process in the bodily mechanism. By injudicious treatment a doctor may do much harm to the patient. Nature's healing may be interfered with or retarded by drugs. Therefore live rationally.

Sri Vasishta said: "Now listen, O Rama, as to the manner in which the two forms of disease, primary and secondary, perish in two ways. The wise say that primary disease has two sub-divisions into the Samanya (ordinary) and the Sara (essential). The former includes the diseases incidental to the body, while the latter the rebirth men are subject to. If the diseases which afflict the body return to their primal source, then they are destroyed. Their primary causes being (bad) thoughts, if these thoughts are destroyed, all bodily diseases will vanish. But the disease of rebirth, coming under the head of Sara, will never perish except through Atma Jnana. Is it possible to suppose that the misconception of a serpent in a rope will be removed except through the discovery of the real rope? But those grievous diseases of the body, which do not arise through the original cause, can be extirpated through Mantras, medicine and the many means proposed by men well-versed in medical lore. I need not expatiate upon this subject any further here."

Here Rama asked Vasishta how mental diseases arise and how they are destroyed. Vasishta thus proceeded: "When the fixed Manas is agitated, then this body also follows in its wake. And when the body is agitated, then there is no proper perception of things that are in one's way, and Prana flies from its proper road like an animal hit by, and reeling under the wound of, an arrow. Through such an agitation Prana instead of pervading the whole body steadily and equally, will vibrate everywhere at an unequal rate. Thereby the Nadis will not maintain a steady position (like electric wires), but will quiver. The food which settles itself down in this body amidst such a commotion is transformed into incurable diseases. Thus through the primary cause (of the mind) is the disease of the body generated. If this primary cause be annihilated at its root, then all diseases will be destroyed. Now hear the path by which diseases may be removed by the uttering of Mantras. Like base gold which, when placed in the crucible, is transmuted through alchemical process into pure gold, the mind is unfailingly rendered pure through true, virtuous and pure actions and through dependence upon the wise. In the mind purified thus, there will thrill unalloyed bliss. Is not the whole world exhilarated with joy when the soft and delicious moon begins to shed its silvery light on it? If the mind becomes purified with the true Sattwa Guna, then Prana Vayu will begin to circulate freely throughout the body, the food taken will be digested properly, and hence no diseases will arise. I have thus described to you the path through which can be destroyed the two kinds of diseases."

CHAPTER III

Importance of Brahmacharya

Brahmacharya is the vow of celibacy in thought, word and deed, by which one attains self-realisation or reaches Brahman. It means control of not only the reproductive indriya (organ) but also the control of all senses in thought, word and deed. The door to Nirvana or perfection is complete Brahmacharya. Complete celibacy is the master-key to open the realms of elysian bliss. The avenue to the abode of supreme peace begins from Brahmacharya or purity.

A Brahmachari is one who is attempting to realise Brahman by his conducting a life of absolute celibacy. Brahmacharya is the conduct of leading a celibate life. "*Yanmanasa Dhayati tad vacha vadati, yad vacha vadati tad karmanan karoti*—That which is thought is spoken by the mouth; that which the mouth speaks the organs of action do." That is the reason why it is said in the Vedas: "*Thanmemanah subha sankalpamastu*—Let my mind think of auspicious things." Entertain sublime divine thoughts. The old evil sexual thoughts will gradually vanish, just as the old nail in a plank is driven by inserting over it a new nail.

"*Brahmacharya Tapasya Deava Mrityupagnata*—The Vedas declare that by Brahmacharya and penance the Devas have conquered death." How did Hanuman become a Mahavir? It is with this weapon of Brahmacharya that he acquired unsurpassable strength and valour. The great Bishma, the grandfather of Pandavas and Kauravas, conquered death by Brahmacharya. It is only Lakshman, the ideal Brahmachari, who put down the man of inestimable prowess, the conqueror of the three worlds Meghanada, son of Ravana. Even Lord Rama could not face him. It is through the force of Brahmacharya that Lakshman was able to defeat that invincible Meghanada. The valour and greatness of emperor Prithviraj was due to the strength of

Brahmacharya. There is nothing in the three worlds that cannot be obtained by a Brahmachari. The Rishis of yore knew fully well of the value of Brahmacharya and that is the reason why they have sung in beautiful verses about its glory and importance.

The Srutis declare: "*Nayam Atma balahinena labhyaha*—This Atma is not attainable by a weak man." In Gita you will find: "*Yadichando Brahmacharyam charanti*—the desiring which Brahmacharya is performed; "*Trividam naraga-syedam dwaram nasanamatmanaha, Kamah krodhascha lobhas tasmatetat, thrayam thyajet*—O Arjuna, triple is the gate of the hell, destructive of the Self; lust, wrath and greed; therefore let man renounce these three." "*Jahi shash-rum mahabaho kamarupam durasidam*—kill this powerful enemy passion by the observance of Brahmacharya."

The fly runs towards the fire or lamp thinking that it is a flower and gets burnt up. Even so the passionate man runs towards a false beautiful form thinking that he can obtain real happiness and gets burnt up in the fire of lust.

Practice of Brahmacharya gives good health, inner strength, peace of mind and a long life. It invigorates the mind and nerves. It helps to conserve physical and mental energy. It augments strength, vigour and vitality. It gives one power to face the difficulties of daily life. A perfect Brahmachari can move the world, and can even command the five elements like Jnana Deva.

Pure water, pure air, wholesome food, physical exercises, outdoor games, walking, rowing, swimming, light games like tennis—all contribute to the maintenance of good health, strength and a high standard of vigour and vitality. There are indeed many ways to gain health and strength. These ways are indispensably requisite. But Brahmacharya is the most important of all. It is the master-key for opening the realms of health and happiness. It is the cornerstone of bliss and unalloyed felicity. It is the only specific that maintains true manliness.

Brahmacharya is the basis for acquiring immortality. It brings material progress and psychic advancement. It is a substratum for a life of peace in Atma. It is a potent weapon for waging war against the internal Asuras, viz., Kama, Khroda, Lobha, etc. It contributes perennial joy, uninterrupted and undecaying bliss. It gives tremendous energy, a clear brain, great will-power, bold understanding, a retentive memory and good Vichara Shakti. Through Brahmacharya and Brahmacharya alone you can have physical, mental and spiritual advancement in life.

Ojas Shakti is spiritual energy that is stored up in the brain. By sublime thoughts, meditation, Japa, worship, Asan and Pranayam practice, the sexual energy can be transmuted into Ojas Shakti and be stored up in the brain. This energy can be utilized for Divine contemplation and spiritual pursuits.

Purity of food brings purity of mind. That power which connects the body and the mind is present in the food that we take. Various kinds of food have various effects on the mind. There are certain kinds of food that make the mind and the body very strong and steady. So it is absolutely essential that we should take pure and Sattwic food. Food has a very close connection with Brahmacharya. If proper attention is given to the purity of food we take, Brahmacharya becomes quite easy.

A glutton can never become a Brahmachari. Control of the tongue is a *sine qua non* if you want to observe Brahmacharya. There is an intimate connection between the tongue and the organ of generation. Tongue is an organ of knowledge. It is born of the Sattwic portion of the water-tanmatra. The organ of generation is an organ of action. It is born of Rajasic portion of the water-tanmatra. They are sister organs as the source is the same. If the tongue is stimulated by Rajasic food, at once the reproductive organ also gets excited. There should be selection and restriction in diet. The food of a Brahmachari must be simple, bland, spiceless, non-irritating and non-stimulating. Moderation in food is also very necessary. Overloading the stomach is highly deleterious. Fruits are highly beneficial. You should take food only when you are really hungry. The stomach will deceive you at times. You may have false hunger; but when you sit down for taking meals, you will have no relish. Dietetic restrictions and fasting are very useful auxiliaries in controlling the carnal mind and in the attainment of Brahmacharya. You should not ignore or make light of them on any account.

The senses are very turbulent. The powerful tubercle bacillus that causes consumption is attacked on all sides by the doctor by various methods like local rubbing, injection, mixtures, powders, etc. So also the senses must be controlled by various methods such as fasting, restriction in diet, Pranayam, Japa, Kirtan, meditation, Pratyahara or abstraction of mind from objects, Dama or self-restraint, Asans, Bandhas, Mudras, thought-control, destruction of Vasanas, etc.

The control of the tongue is a *sine qua non* if you want to control lust. The tongue must be controlled first. Then it will be easy to control passion. Delicious Rajasic foods excite the organ of generation.

One drop of semen is manufactured out of 40 drops of blood according to medical science. According to the Ayurveda, it is elaborated out of 80 drops of blood. Just as sugar is all-pervading in the sugarcane, butter in milk, so also semen pervades the whole body. Just as buttermilk is thin after the butter has been removed, so also semen is thinned by its wastage. The more the wastage of semen, the greater the weakness. In Yoga Shastras it is said: "*Maranam bindu patanat jivanam bindu rakshanat*—falling of semen brings death; preservation of semen gives life." Semen is the real vitality of men. It is the hidden treasure for man. It imparts Brahma Tejas to the face and strength to the intellect.

If the spermatic secretion in men is continuous, it must either be expelled or reabsorbed. As a result of the most patient and persevering scientific investigations, it has been found that whenever the seminal secretions are conserved and thereby reabsorbed into the system, it goes towards enriching the blood and strengthening the brain. Dr. Dio Louis taught that the conservation of this element is essential to strength of body, vigour of mankind and keeness of intellect. strength of body, vigour of mankind and keenness of intellect.

Another writer, Dr. E. P. Miller, says: "All wastes of spermatic secretions, either voluntary or involuntary, is a direct waste of life force. It is almost universally conceded that the choicest elements of the blood enter into the composition of the spermatic secretion. If these conclusions are correct, then it follows that a chaste life is essential to man's well being."

Just as oil is sucked up by a wick and burns with glowing light, so also the Veerya or semen flows up by the practice of Yoga Sadhana and is converted into Tejas or Ojas. The Brahmachari shines with Brahmic aura in his face. Brahmacharya is the bright light that shines in the house of human body. It is the fully blossomed flower of life around which bees of strength, patience, knowledge, purity and Dhriti wander about humming hither and thither. In other words, he who observes Brahmacharya will be endowed with the above qualities. The Hindu Scriptures declare emphatically: "*Ayastheto balam veeryam prapana seerscha; Punyam cha sat pariyatwam cha vardhayet Brahmacharyaya*—By the practice of Brahmacharya, longevity, glory, strength, vigour, knowledge, wealth, undecaying fame, virtues, devotion to Truth increase."

Regular meditation and Japa of Mantra, Sattwic food, Sat Sangha (association with Sadhus, wise and great men), practice of Pranayam, Asans, study of religious books, Vichara or the enquiry into the nature of Atma Self or "who am I?" seclusion, will entirely annihilate lust, however powerful the old Samskaras and Vasanas may be. Positive always overcomes negative. You need not be discouraged at any rate. Plunge yourself seriously in Yogic practice, kill this Mara and come out victorious in the struggle. Shine as a brilliant Yogi.

Blessed is the Brahmachari who has taken the vow of celibacy for the whole life. Twice blessed is that Brahmachari who is sincerely struggling to destroy lust and attain perfect purity. Thrice blessed is that Brahmachari who has completely rooted out lust and has attained Self-realisation. Glory to such exalted Brahmacharis! They are veritable Gods on the earth. May their blessings be upon you all!

PART SECOND

COURSE OF YOGIC EXERCISES

FIFTEEN MINUTES DAILY

(For all-round development)

	Pranayam	*Minutes*
1.	Sukh Purvak or Ujjayi or Bhastrika	4
2.	Sitali	1
	Poses	
3.	Paschimottanasan or Padahasthasan or Ardhamatsyendrasan or Trikonasan ...	2
4.	Salabhasan or Dhanurasan or Bhujangasan	2
5.	Sarvangasan and Matsyasan or Sirshasan ...	2
6.	Nauli or Uddiyana	2
7.	Yoga Mudra	1
8.	Savasan	1
	Minutes	15

First practise the poses and then Pranayam. Savasan should be done at the end of the course. The meditative poses can be practised during Japa and meditation. To maintain the elasticity of the spine it is necessary that the spine should be pulled posteriorly, anteriorly, sideways and twisted too. All the organs, muscles and nerves should be toned up. The above set of Asans if practised daily for fifteen minutes will bestow on the practitioner everlasting youth, happiness, energy and a high standard of vigour and vitality.

CHAPTER I

Yogic Exercises

MEDITATIVE POSES

Yogic Culture is divided into eight Angas (limbs or steps), viz., Yama, Niyama, Asan, Pranayam, Pratyahara, Dharana, Dhyana and Samadhi. Yama is the practice of Ahimsa (non-killing or non-injuring), Satya (truthfulness), Asteya (non-stealing), Brahmacharya (celibacy), Aparigraha (abstinence from greed). Niyama is the practice of Saucha (internal and external purity), Santos (contentment), Tapas (mortification), Swadhyaya (study of scriptures), Ishwara-pranidhana (self-surrender). Asan is the third Anga. If you want to enjoy the full spiritual benefits of Asans, you must first practise well the first two steps, Yama and Niyama.

Asans can be divided into two broad divisions, viz., meditative poses and poses for health and strength. According to Yoga Shastras there are four excellent meditative poses: Padmasan, Siddhasan, Swastikasan and Sukhasan.

You must be able to sit in one of these four Asans at a stretch for full three hours without shaking the body. Without securing a steady Asan, you cannot get on well in meditation. The more steady you are in your Asan, the more you will be able to concentrate and make your mind one-pointed.

Select any one of the four that is suitable to you and sit for fifteen minutes and gradually increase the period to three hours. When you sit on the Asan, keep the head, neck and trunk in one straight line. Do not bend the back.

When you sit for meditation in the Asan, close your eyes and gently concentrate on Trikute (the space between the two eyebrows). Tip of the nose, Anahata Chakra (the lotus of the heart) are other places for concentration.

1. PADMASAN

This is one of the most important poses. When Padmasan is demonstrated, it gives the appearance of a lotus. In Sanskrit Padma means lotus. The two feet on the opposite thighs represent the petals of a lotus.

Amongst the four poses prescribed for meditation, Padmasan comes foremost. It is the best Asan for contemplation. Rishis like Gheranda, Sandilya and others speak very highly of this vital Asan. It is suitable for householders, men and women.

TECHNIQUE

These four Asans, viz., Padmasan, Siddhasan, Swastikasan and Sukhasan, are practised for Japa and meditation. In your meditation room, in front of the picture of your Ishta Devata or Guru, spread a Kusa seat (seat made of Kusa grass) and over this a deer or tiger skin. You can spread a piece of cotton cloth on this deer or tiger skin and then sit for meditation. Or spread on the ground a four-folded blanket and over this a cloth. This also will serve you well.

Sit on this seat and stretch the legs forward. Take hold of the right foot with the two hands and folding the leg at the knee, place the foot on the left thigh. Similarly fold the left leg and place it on the right thigh. Keep the body erect and place the hands between the heels, one over the other. If this is not suitable to you, you can keep the hands on the knees. The left knee or thigh should not be raised from the ground.

These meditative poses are highly suitable for Japa and contemplative purposes. They increase the digestive fire and give good appetite, health and happiness. They remove rheumatism. They keep the wind, bile and phlegm in proper proportions. They purify and strengthen the nerves of the legs and thighs. They are suitable for keeping up Brahmacharya (celibacy).

2. SIDDHASAN

"Siddha" means an adept in Sanskrit. Since great adepts used this Asan, it bears the name Siddhasan. Siddhas (perfected Yogins) speak very highly to this Asan. Young Brahmacharins and those who attempt to get established in celibacy should practise this Asan.

Sit on your seat. Stretch the legs forward. Bend the left leg at the knee and place the heel at the soft portion of the perineum, the space between the anus and the scrotum. Then fold the right leg and place the heel against the pubic bone or just above the genitals. The genitals should be nicely arranged in such a manner that no pressure is felt. Keep the body erect and place the hands as in Padmasan.

3. SWASTIKASAN

"Swastika" means 'prosperous' in Sanskrit. This Asan brings prosperity and success to the practitioner. Hence this pose bears the name Swastikasan.

Sit on the seat. Stretch the legs. Bend the right leg at the knee and keep the heel against the groin of the left thigh so that the sole will be lying in close touch with the thigh. Similarly bend the left leg and set it against the right groin. Insert the toes of the left leg between the right calf and thigh muscles. Now you will find the two feet between the calf and thigh muscles. This is very comfortable for meditation. Keep the hands as instructed in Padmasan.

4. SUKHASAN

An easy, comfortable posture for Japa and meditation is Sukhasan, the important point being the head, neck and the trunk should be in a line without any curve.

5. SIRSHASAN

In Sanskrit 'Sirsh' means head. As you have to stand in this Asan on your head in a topsy-turvy manner, it is called Sirshasan. The practitioner gets the maximum physical and spiritual benefits through this Asan. So this is the most important one. This is the King of all Asans.

Technique

The skull has to bear the whole weight of the body in this Asan. You should use a soft cushion or a four-folded

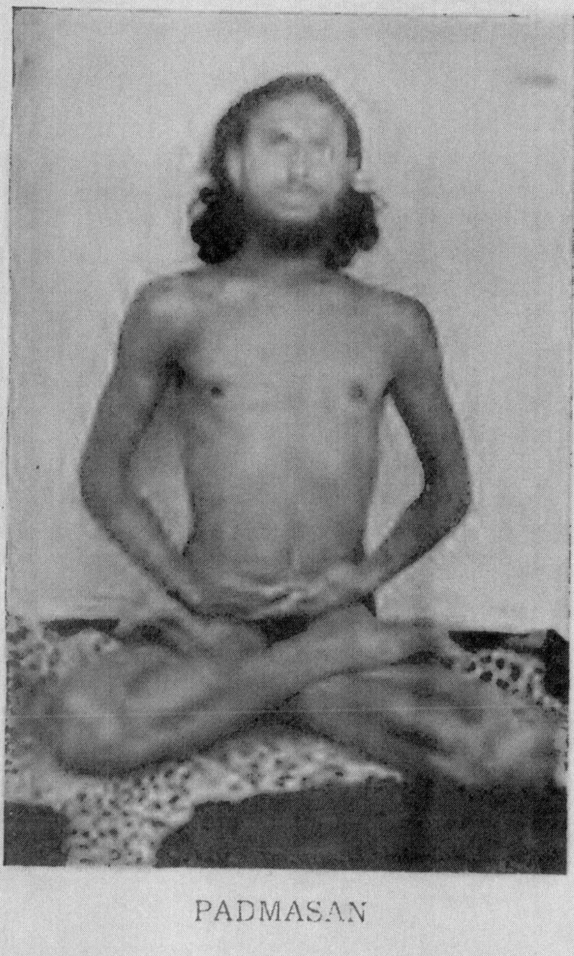

PADMASAN

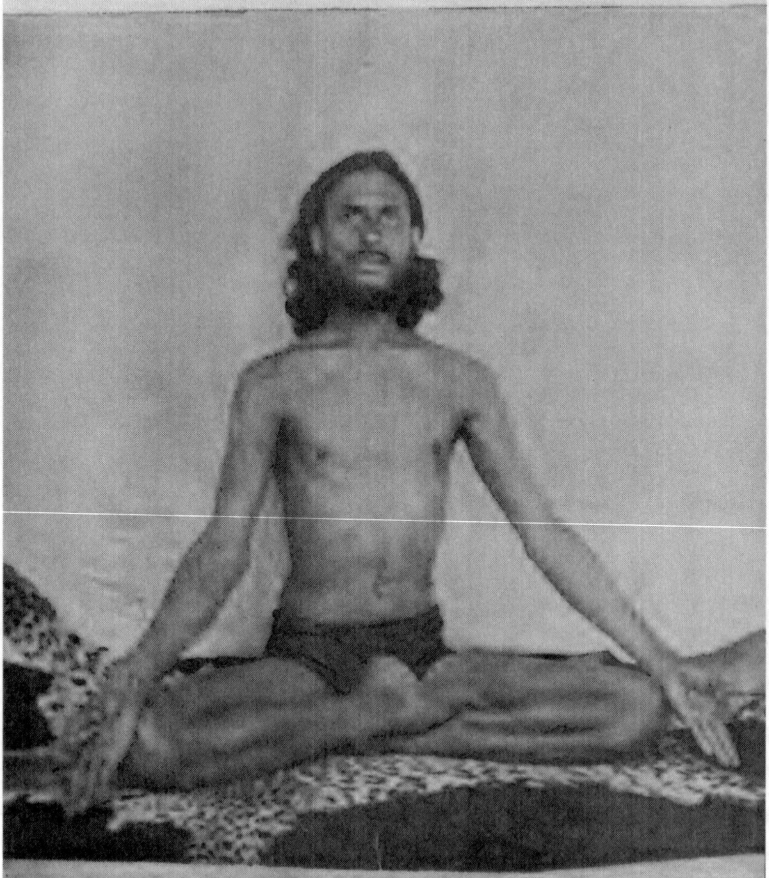

SIDDHASAN

blanket. Spread the blanket on the ground. Sit on the knees. By interweaving the fingers make a finger-lock and keep it on the carpet in such a way that the locked hands serve as a vertex and the two elbows as the base enabling the forearms to balance the body. The top of the head may be supported from behind by the finger-lock while doing this Asan.

Then keep the top of your head on the carpet close to the finger-lock. The parietal (frontal) portion of the top of the head should be placed on the carpet and not the portion nearer to the forehead. This will help you to keep the spine erect in this Asan. If the portion nearer to the forehead is used, the spine will suffer a curvature in balancing the whole body.

Now the knees are brought close to the body and the toes allowed to touch the ground for balancing. When the trunk is sufficiently thrown back you can slowly remove the toes from the ground. Slowly raise the legs high up in the air till the whole body becomes erect. Stand in the Asan for five seconds only and gradually increase the period to half an hour. In well-regulated systematic Asan exercises, even five minutes will be quite sufficient to derive the maximum benefits. Always breathe through the nose only and never through the mouth. In the beginning for a few days you will find difficulty in breathing through the nose. In a few days, this trouble will pass away.

In learning the Asan in the above manner, you will not require any help. You yourself can learn the method of balancing by repeated attempts. Instead of a finger-lock method, you can keep the palms of your hands on the ground one on each side. You will find this quite easy. When you have learnt to balance the whole body, you can take to the finger-lock method. Or you can take the help of a wall. Try to remove the legs from the wall. Or you may ask a friend to support the legs and to leave you when you have learnt how to balance yourself.

Bring the legs slowly to the ground to the original position. Lower the legs very, very slowly and avoid jerks. After completing the Asan stand erect for a minute or two. This will harmonise the circulation of blood.

BENEFITS

In this pose the whole body is inverted. Owing to gravitation, the arch of the aorta, the common carotids, the innominate and the subclavian are flooded with rich arterial blood and in this Asan alone can the brain draw a rich supply of pure blood. The importance of the brain, the root of all nerves, can be very well understood from the Chapter: "Brain and Nerves." The 12 pairs of cranial nerves, the spinal cord, the 31 pairs of the spinal nerves and the sympathetic system get sufficient nourishment. All the defects of the nerves, eyes, nose, throat and ears are completely removed by the practice of this Asan. It is a powerful nervine tonic. The whole nervous system is nourished and toned. All the venous blood that has to rise against gravity is now helped by the force of gravity and so the veins and their valves get ample rest. So this Asan will serve as a cure for varicose-veins.

This is extremely useful in keeping up Brahmacharya. The seminal energy is transmuted into Ojas Shakti. This is called a sex-sublimation. Persons suffering from wet-dreams or Spermatorrhoea will derive very great benefit from this Asan. The seminal energy is converted into Ojas Shakti and flows towards the brain so that it may be stored up as a spiritual force which may be used for a contemplative purpose, Dhyana.

Sirshasan invigorates, energises and vivifies. It is a panacea (cure-all) for all human ailments. It is a powerful blood purifier. It cures all the diseases of the liver, spleen, lungs and the genito-urinary system. It cures renal colic, deafness, diabetes, piles, pyorrhoea and constipation. The digestive power will improve. This Asan is best suited for ladies also Many uterine and ovarian diseases are cured. It is not advisable for ladies to practise this Asan during the monthly periods and pregnancy.

Sterility disappears. Memory improves admirably. Lawyers, occultists and thinkers will find it extremely useful. It

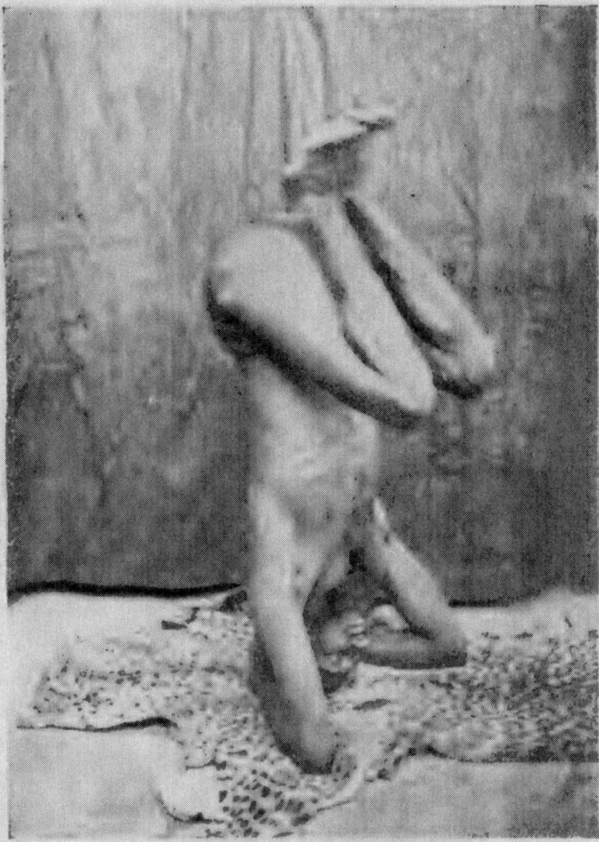

SIRSHASAN (Second Stage)

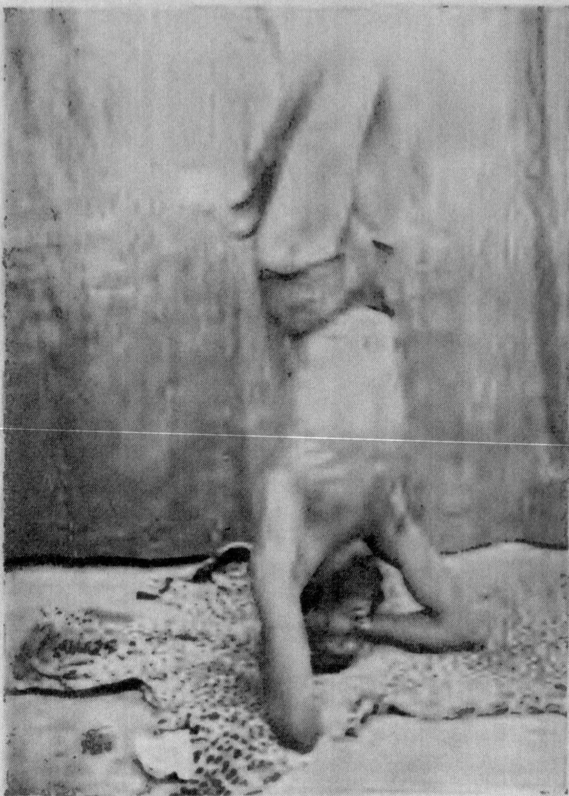

SIRSHASAN (Third Stage)

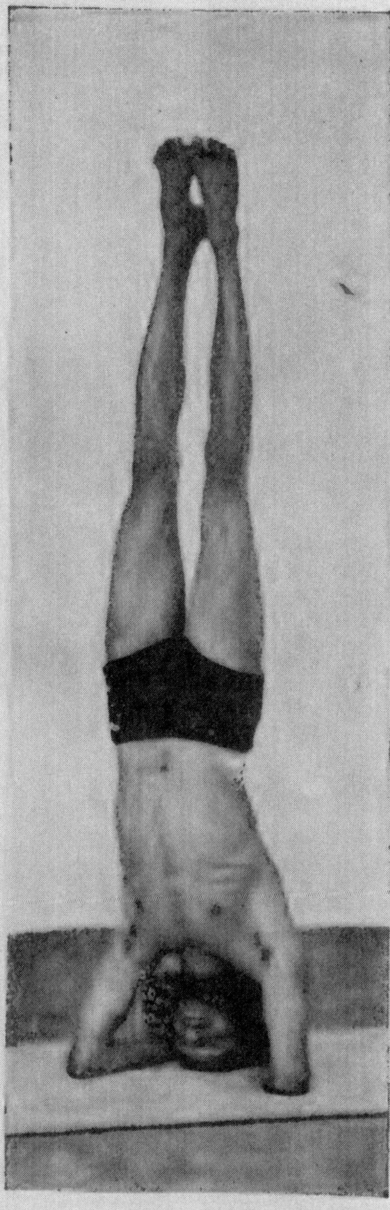

SIRSHASAN (Final Stage)

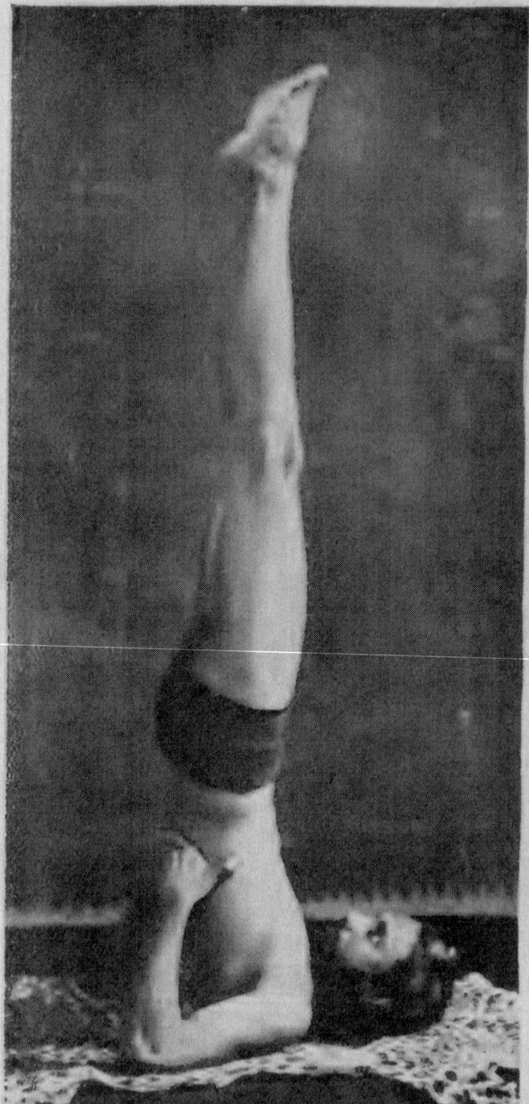

SARVANGASAN

you observe the breath, you will notice that it becomes finer and finer. This Asan leads to natural Pranayam and helps in awakening Kundalini Shakti that lies dormant in the Muladhara Chakra or basal Lotus.

6. SARVANGASAN

"Sarvang" means 'all parts.' So the very name suggests that this pose is concerned with all the parts of the body. It is one of the unique poses which rejuvenates the whole system.

TECHNIQUE

Spread a thick blanket on the ground. Lie quite flat on the back. Slowly raise the legs. Lift the trunk, hips and legs quite vertical. Rest the elbows on the ground firmly and support the back with the two hands. Raise the legs till they become quite vertical. Press the chin against the chest. This is the chin-lock. While you perform this Asan the back of the neck, the posterior part of the head and the shoulders should touch the ground. Breathe slowly and concentrate on the thyroid glands which are situated in the neck. Do not allow the body to shake to and fro. When the Asan is over, lower the legs very slowly and with elegance. Avoid jerks. Do the Asan very gracefully. In this Asan the whole weight of the body is thrown on the shoulders. You can do this Asan twice daily, morning and evening. Immediately after performing this Asan, you will have to do Matsyasan to derive the full benefit from it. Remain in this Asan for two minutes and gradually increase the period to 30 minutes.

Just as Sirshasan is intended to tone up the whole nervous system, this easy and wonderful Asan is intended to promote the secretion of the thyroids and through it the whole body and all its functions. The thyroids are the most important glands of the endocrine system. In this Asan the thyroid glands receive rich supply of blood. Healthy thyroids mean healthy functioning of the circulatory, respiratory, alimentary and genito-urinary systems of the body.

This Asan is a good substitute for modern thyroid treatment. It cures the dreadful leprosy. The patient will have to live on milk during the whole period of treatment. Milk helps the thyroid to secrete its juice in sufficient quantity to help the economy of nature in its restorative function and regeneration. If the patient takes a sun bath morning and evening, his recovery will be hastened.

This Asan keeps back the ravages of old age and keeps a man young always. Those young men who have lost weight of the testes owing to bad habits like masturbation, sexual excesses, etc., will retain the weight by this Asan. They can combine Uddiyana Bandha and Nauli Kriya and regain their lost vitality and energy.

Sarvangasan cures dyspepsia, constipation, appendicitis, other gastro-intestinal disorders and varicose-veins. It supplies a large quantity of blood to the spinal roots of the nerves. It is this Asan which centralises the blood in the spinal column and nourishes it beneficially. Except through this Asan, the nerve roots cannot receive an adequate blood supply. It keeps the spine quite elastic. Elasticity of the spine means everlasting youth. It prevents the bone from early ossification (hardening). Sarvangasan awakens Kundalini and augments the digestive power.

7. MATSYASAN

In Sanskrit "Matsya" means a fish. A person can float on water, without swimming for a long time like a fish.

Technique

Spread a blanket on the ground and sit on it with the legs stretched. Bend the right leg and place the heel on the left hip joint. Again bend the left leg and place the heel on the right hip joint. This is Padmasan or foot-lock.

Then lie on the back. The Padmasan should not be raised from the ground. Rest the elbows or hands on the ground. Now lift the trunk and head. Rest the top of the head on the ground by bending the back well and throwing the neck well behind. Then catch hold of the toes. This is Matsyasan. It is performed immediately after Sarvangasan. Remain in this Asan for 2 or 3 minutes.

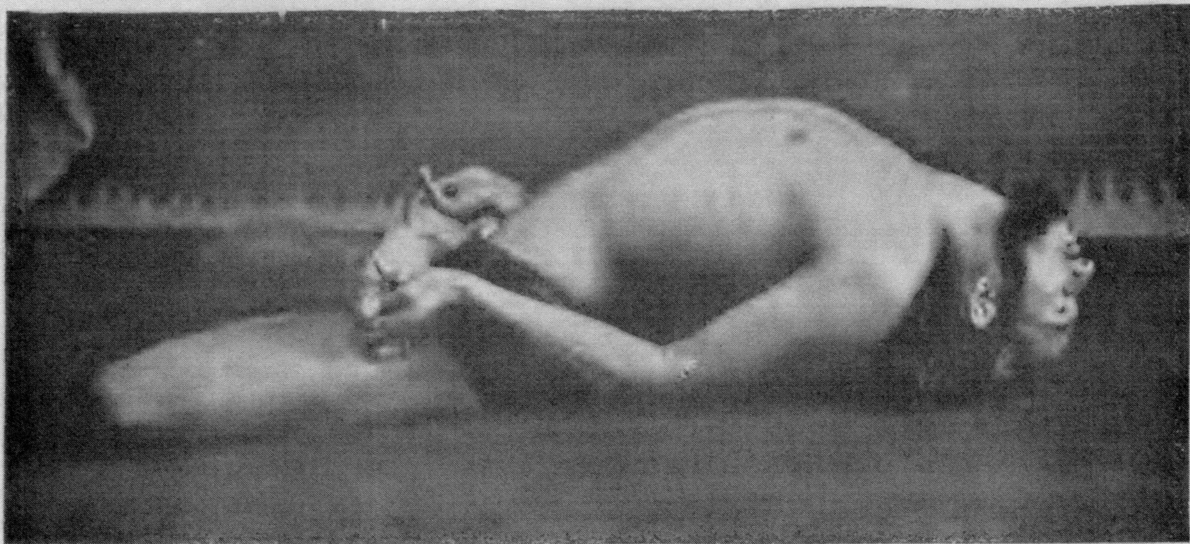

MATSYASAN

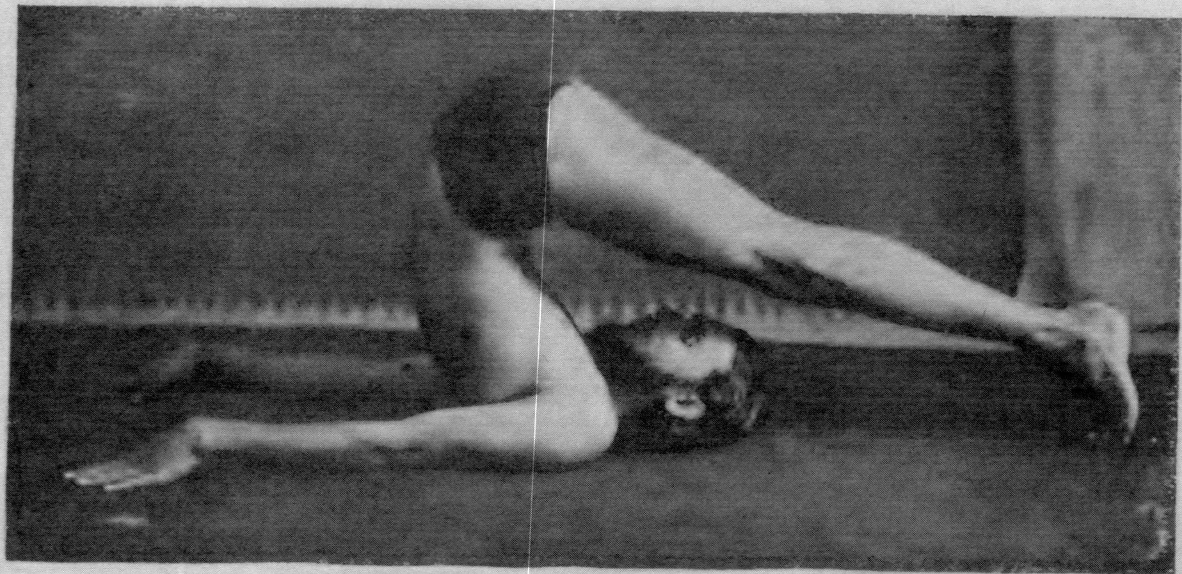

HALASAN

Those fatty persons who find it difficult to form a foot-lock, may simply bend the legs at the knees and so practise it.

Benefits

This Asan relieves the crampness and stiffness in the neck caused by Sarvangasan. Matsyasan naturally massages the congested parts of the neck and shoulders. In Sarvangasan the neck is bent well forwards whereas in Matsyasan the neck is bent backwards.

In Matsyasan also the thyroids and para-thyroids receive plenty of blood. The waist, the back and the neck will grow strong. In this Asan the practitioner can breathe freely and deeply, as the larynx or wind-box and trachea or windpipe are thrown open widely. The apices of the lungs which are located just behind and above the clavicular bone or collar bone in common parlance, receive a proper amount of fresh air and a sufficient supply of pure oxygen. The cervical and upper dorsal nerves are nourished with a good quantity of blood and so toned up properly. The endocrine glands, and the pituitary and pineal glands that are located in the brain are also stimulated and toned up. These glands play a vital part in the physiological functioning of the various systems of the body. In this pose the abdominal muscles are exercised. So this Asan removes constipation and massages the abdominal viscera or ograns.

8. HALASAN

On completion this pose gives the exact appearance of a plough. Hala means a 'plough.'

Lie flat on your back on a carpet. Keep the two hands near the thighs, the palms towards the ground. Without bending the legs, slowly raise them higher up. Do not raise the hands but raise the hips and the lumbar part of the back also and bring down the legs till the toes touch the ground beyond the head. Keep the knees quite straight and close together. The legs and thighs must be in one straight line. Press the chin against the chest. Breathe slowly through the nose. This is Sarvangasan. Remain in this Asan for two minutes. Then slowly raise the legs and bring them to the original position of lying on the ground flat.

There is a better variety of this Asan. When the toes reach the ground, remove the hands and catch hold of the toes. The pose can be repeated 3 to 6 times with advantage. For attaining spiritual benefits, the pose should be maintained for a long time at a stretch.

Benefits

In Bhujang, Salabh and Dhanurasan the deep and superficial muscles of the back are contracted and relaxed, but in Halasan these muscles are fully stretched and relaxed. These muscles of the back are responsible for the healthy condition of the spine. The abdominal muscles contract vigorously and become very strong. The whole spine is steadily pulled posteriorly. Every vertebra and ligament that is attached to it receive plenty of blood and become healthy. All the 31 pairs of spinal nerves and the sympathetic system are well nourished by a copious blood supply and so are toned up. This Asan prevents the early ossification of the vertebral bones. He who practises this Asan is very nimble, agile and full of energy. Various sorts of myalgia, lumbago, sprain in the neck, neuralgia, etc., are cured. Obesity or corpulence and habitual or chronic constipation, gulma (chronic dyspepsia), liver and spleen complaints are also cured.

9. SALABHASAN

"Salabha" means a 'locust' in Sanskrit. When the pose is demonstrated, it gives the appearance of a locust with its tail raised.

Technique

Lie prone (on the face) on the blanket and keep the hands alongside the body, palms facing upwards. Rest the chin on the ground by raising the head a little higher up or rest

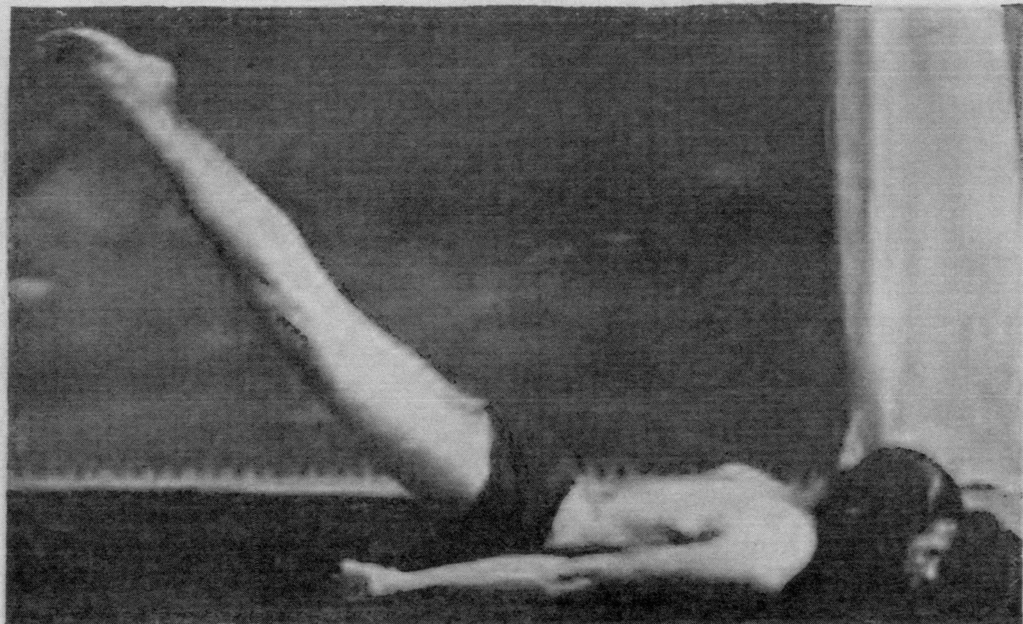

SALABHASAN

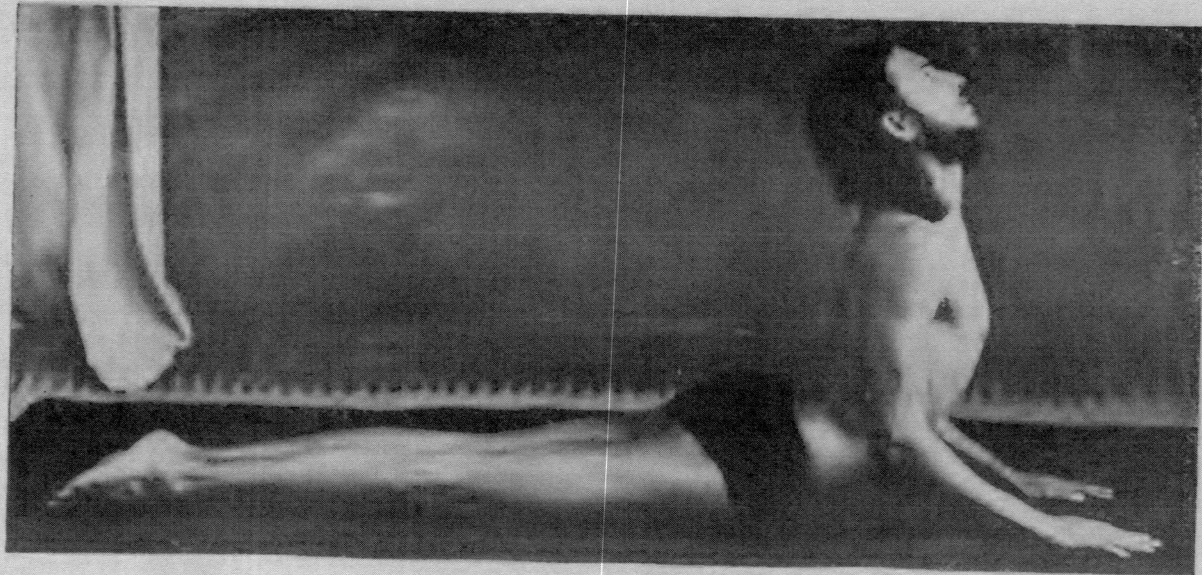

BHUJANGASAN

the chin, the mouth and the nose on the ground. Now inhale slowly. Stiffen the whole body and raise the legs high. The knees should be kept straight. The sacrum too should be raised a little along with the legs. Now the chest and the hands will feel the burden of the legs. Keep the thighs, legs and toes in a straight line. Remain in the pose for 20 seconds and slowly bring down the legs, and then exhale slowly. Repeat the process 3 or 4 times according to your capacity. Do not go so far as to induce fatigue. Bhujangasan exercises the upper part of the body and Salabhasan the lower extremity of the body.

Benefits

The intra-abdominal pressure is increased to a very high degree. It relieves constipation and tones up the liver, pancreas and kidneys. All the abdominal muscles are strengthened to a very great degree. The vertebra of the lumbar and the sacrum bone also get toned up. The sacral, coccygeal and the lower part of the lumbar regions receive plenty of blood and so become healthy and strong. Owing to the Kumbhak done during this pose, the lungs expand and become strong.

10. BHUJANGASAN

When this Asan is fully done, it gives the appearance of a hooded cobra. The raised trunk, neck and head represent the hood. Hence the significant name. 'Bhujang' means a cobra in Sanskrit.

Technique

Lie down on the blanket keeping the back above. Relax all the muscles completely. Place the palms below the corresponding shoulders on the blanket. Raise the head and upper portion of the body slowly just as the cobra raises its hood. Bend the spine well. Do not raise the body suddenly with a jerk. Raise it little by little so that you can actually feel the bending of the vertebrae one by one and the pressure travelling downwards from the cervical, dorsal and lumbar regions and lastly to the sacral regions. Let the body from the navel downwards to the toes touch the ground. Retain the posture for a minute and slowly bring down the head little by little. You may repeat the process 6 times.

Benefits

All the Western physical culturists unanimously acclaim the importance of rendering the spine supple and elastic. Elasticity of the spine means health, vitality and youth to the individual. The deep and superficial muscles of the back are well toned up. This pose relieves the pain in the back that may have been caused due to overwork. The abdominal muscles are pulled and thereby strengthened. The intra-abdominal pressure is increased to a very high degree and so constipation is removed. The whole abdominal viscera are toned up. Every vertebra and its ligaments are pulled backwards and they get a rich blood supply. It increases bodily heat and destroys a host of ailments. It gives good appetite.

Bhujangasan is particularly useful for ladies in toning up their ovaries and uterus. It is a powerful tonic. It will relieve amenorrhoea, dysmenorrhoea, leucorrhoea and various other utero-ovarine troubles.

11. DHANURASAN

When this Asan is performed, it gives the appearance of a bow. Dhanur means a bow. The stretched hands and legs represent the string of a bow; and the body and the thighs represent the bow proper.

Technique

Lie prone on the blanket. Relax the muscles. Now bend the legs over the thighs. Catch hold of the right ankle with the right hand and the left ankle with the left hand firmly. Raise the head, body and the knees by tugging at the legs with the hands so that the whole burden of the body rests on the abdomen and the spine is nicely arched backwards like a bow.

Maintain this pose for a few seconds and then relax the body. You can either make a Kumbhak or breathe normally. Even weak persons can do this Asan easily. To perform

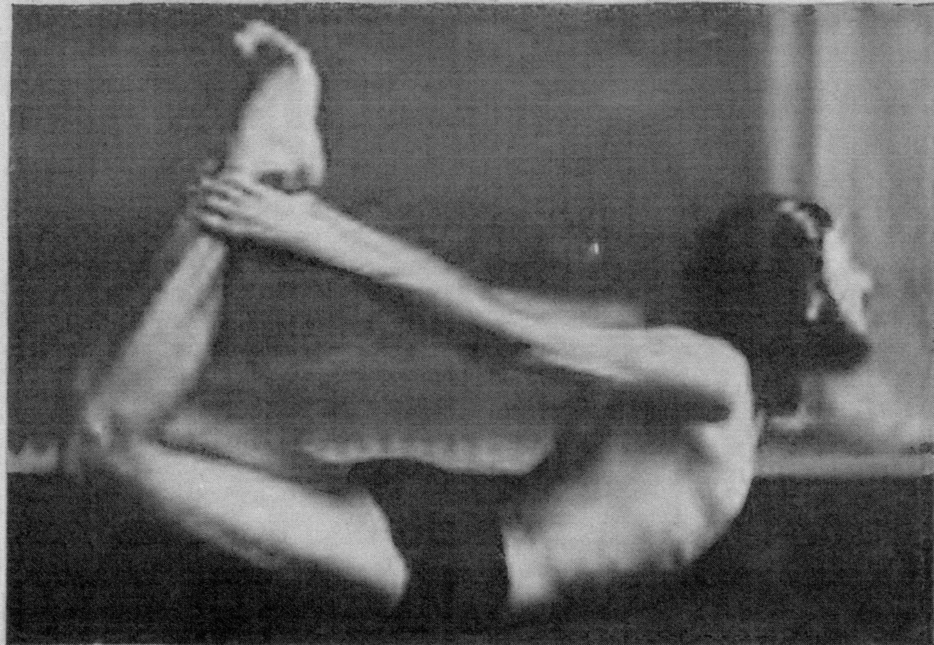

DHANURASAN

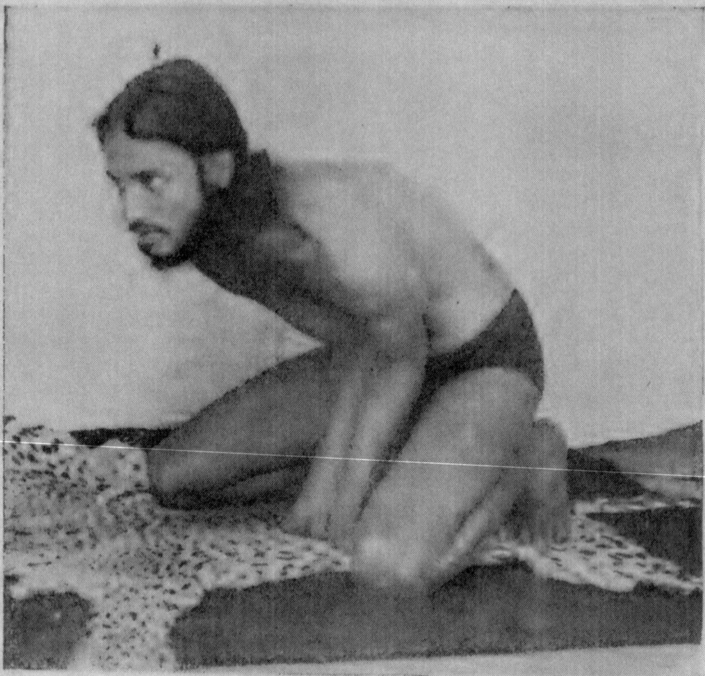

MAYURASAN (First Stage)

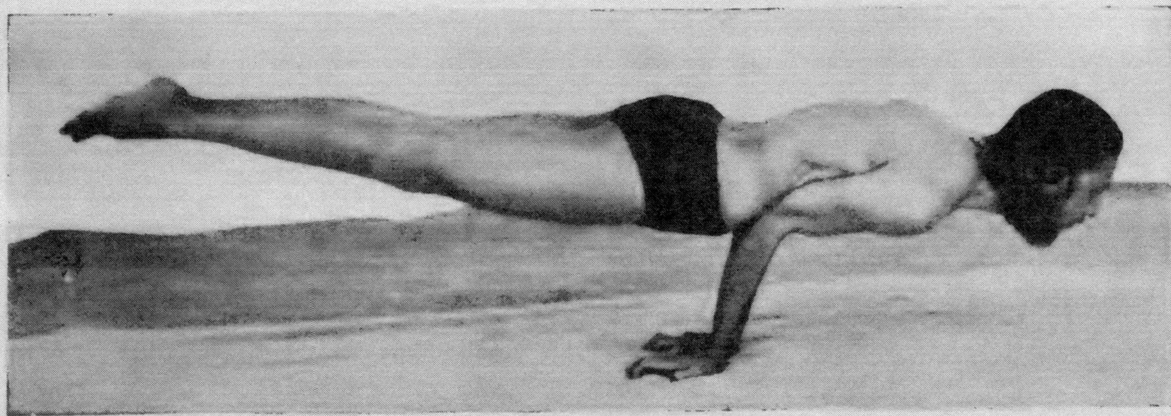

MAYURASAN (Final Stage)

the Asan a sudden movement of the body is required. Be steady. Do not jerk the body.

Dhanurasan complements or supplements Bhujangasan. We can say it is a combination of Bhujang and Salabhasan with the addition of catching the ankles. Bhujang, Salabh and Dhanur Asans form a valuable combination. They always go together. They form one set of Asans. Dhanurasan should be repeated 3 or 4 times.

BENEFITS

The very appearance of the pose gives one the idea that it is a combination of Bhujangasan and Salabhasan. All the benefits of Salabh and Bhujangasans can be derived to a greater degree in Dhanurasan. The back muscles are well massaged. This removes constipation and cures dyspepsia, rheumatism and gastro-intestinal disorders. It reduces fat, energises digestion, invigorates appetite and relieves congestion of the blood in the abdominal viscera. This Asan is highly suitable for ladies.

12. MAYURASAN

In Sanskrit "Mayur" means peacock. When this Asan is exhibited the body resembles a peacock which has *spread out* its bundle of feathers at the back.

TECHNIQUE

Kneel on a blanket. Join the two arms together and rest them on the ground, palms turned down. You may curve the fingers slightly. This facilitates balancing. Keep the hands firm. Now you have steady and firm forearms for supporting the whole body. Bring down the abdomen slowly against the conjoined elbows. Support your body on your elbows. Then stretch your legs. Inhale and raise the legs together from the ground. Raise the legs straight on a level with the head, parallel to the ground. Keep the posture steady for 5 seconds and then rest the toes on the ground and exhale. This is Mayurasan. Rest for a few minutes.

BENEFITS

This is the best Asan known for all stomach disorders. Owing to the pressure of hands on the stomach below the navel, the abdominal aorta is partially compressed and the blood that is thus checked is directed towards the digestive organs. The liver, pancreas, stomach, kidneys are toned up. The intra-abdominal pressure is increased to a very high degree and the abdominal viscera is toned up. Mayurasan awakens the Kundalini Shakti.

Mayurasan has got a charm of its own. It braces you up quickly. It serves like a hypodermic injection of adrenalin or digitalin. This is a wonderful Asan for improving digestion. Sluggishness of the liver or hepatic torpidity disappears. This one Asan can give you maximum benefit in a minimum space of time; a few seconds daily are enough.

13. ARDHA-MATSYENDRASAN

"Ardha" means half. This is half of Matsyendrasan. This Asan takes its name from the Rishi or Yogi Matsyendra, who first taught this Asan to the students of Hatha Yoga.

Technique

Spread a blanket on the ground and sit on it with the legs stretched out. Bend the right leg at the knee and set the heel against the perineum. Do not allow the heel to move from this space. Now bend the left leg at the knee and with the help of the hands arrange the foot to rest on the ground by the external side of the right thigh. Then passing the right hand over the left knee, catch hold of the left foot firmly by the right hand. The left knee is now placed at the right axilla. In order to have more mechanical advantage for twisting the spine, the left hand is now swung back and the right thigh is caught. Now steadily pull and twist the spine. To help the spine to twist evenly all through, the neck too is turned towards the left shoulder. Keep the chest erect and forwards. Remain in this pose for 5 seconds. Then release the hands and legs. Repeat the same process, twisting the spine on the right side by changing the limbs, thus accomplishing the twist on both sides. This will complete the whole spinal twist.

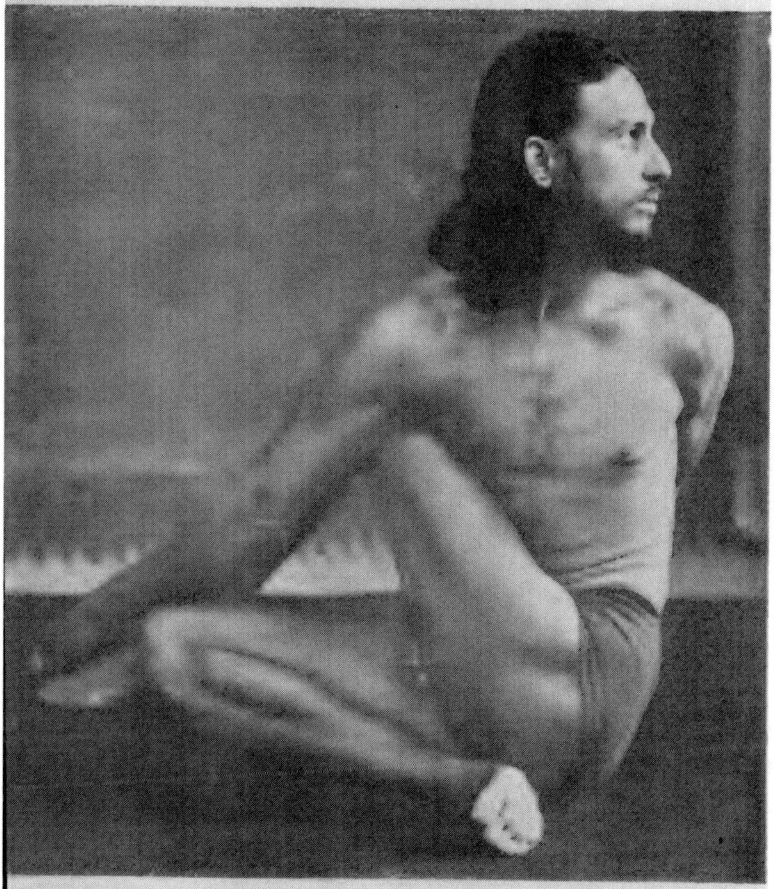

ARDHAMATSYENDRASAN

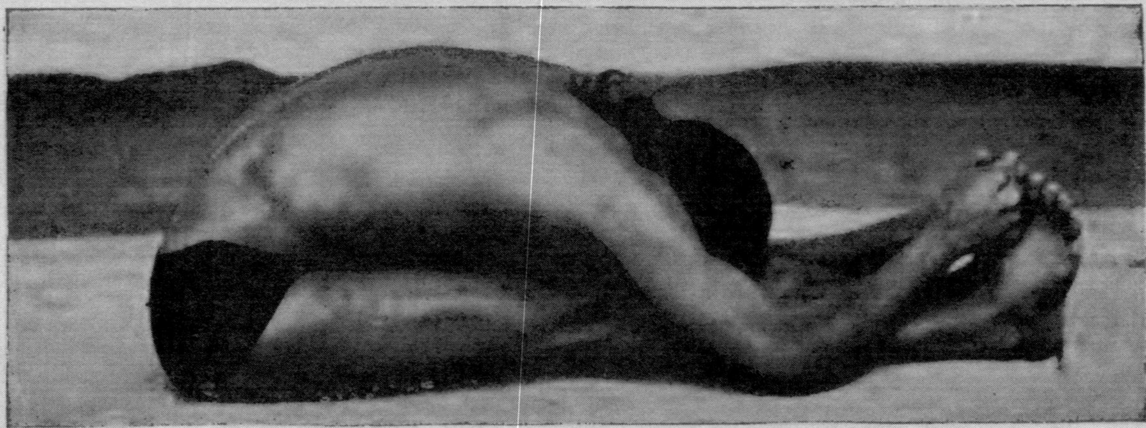

PASCHIMOTTANASAN

Benefits

Ardha-matsyendrasan keeps the spine elastic and well massages the abdominal organs. Lumbago and all sorts of muscular rheumatism of the back muscles are cured. The spinal nerve-roots and the sympathetic system are toned up. They draw a good supply of blood. This is a very good Asan for constipation and dyspepsia. In this Asan every vertebra is rotated on both sides. The ligaments too that are attached to the vertebra get this movement and so receive the rich supply of blood. All the spinal nerves are toned up. The Asan gives lateral movement to the spine to a great extent.

14. PASCHIMOTTANASAN

Lie flat on the back (supine) on the carpet. Keep the legs and thighs fixed to the ground. Stiffen your body. Slowly raise the head and chest and assume a sitting pose. Now exhale and bend yourself further till you are able to catch hold of your toes. You may even bury your face between the knees. Remain thus for 5 seconds and then slowly raise the body and resume the supine position. You should now inhale. Repeat this Asan 3 or 4 times.

Benefits

This is an excellent Asan. It makes the breath flow through the Brahma Nadi or Sushumna Nadi and rouses the gastric fire. All the abdominal muscles get vigorously contracted. This is a powerful abdominal exercise. This Asan stimulates the abdominal viscera such as the kidneys, liver, pancreas. It cures piles and diabetes. This Asan is a good preventive of nocturnal emissions. It is a very good Asan for stretching the posterior muscles of the body. The hamstring muscles at the back of the knees are strengthened. The epigastric nerves, the bladder, the prostrate, the lumbar nerves and the sympathetic are all toned up and kept in a sound condition. The spine becomes elastic and thereby perennial youth is established. Halasan and Paschimottan-asan bend the spine anteriorly, in a perfect manner.

15. PADAHASTHASAN

This can be styled as "Standing Paschimottanasan." In Sanskrit "Pada" means 'feet' and "Hastha" means 'legs.'

Technique

Stand erect. Raise your hands over your head and inhale deeply. Then exhale slowly and while exhaling bend the body till the hands reach the toes and the nose touches the knees. The raised hands should be in contact with the ears all throughout, even while bending the body. After a little practice you will be able to bury the face between the knees and keep the palms firmly on the ground. Remain in this pose for 5 seconds. Then slowly raise your body and come to the standing position. When you raise your body, you should inhale slowly. Repeat this pose 4 times.

Benefits

All the benefits of Paschimottanasan are derived from this Asan. The spine becomes supple and is lengthened. It is also an excellent exercise for increasing your height. The adipose tissue on the abdomen will disappear. This Asan is very suitable for ladies for reducing any excess of fat and for developing a graceful figure. You will feel much invigorated after performing this Asan. The body will be rendered light.

16. TRIKONASAN

"Trikona" means "triangle." Since this Asan when demonstrated gives the appearance of a triangle, it bears the name Trikonasan.

Technique

Stand erect keeping the feet two or three feet apart. Now stretch your arms wide on the sides in a line with the shoulders. The palms should fall downward. Bend to the left slowly and touch the left toes with your left hand. Remain thus for 5 seconds and slowly return to your standing position. Do not bend your legs or hands when you bend down or when you get up. From the standing position bend

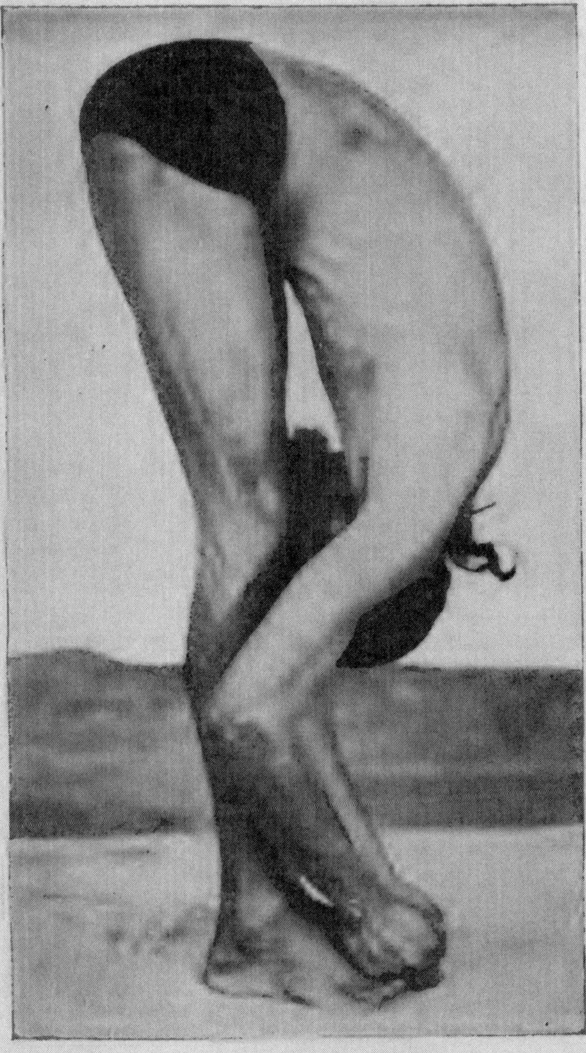

PADAHASTHASAN

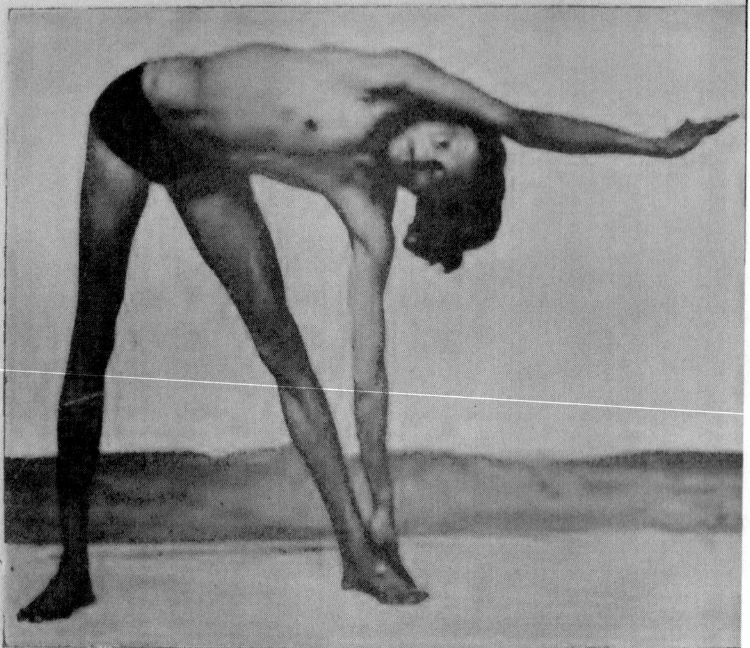

TRIKONASAN

to your right next and touch your right toes with the right hand. Remain for 5 seconds in this position and then come back to your original standing position. Repeat thus 4 times. This is Trikonasan.

Benefits

Trikonasan tones up the spinal nerves and the abdominal organs, increases peristalsis of the bowels and invigorates the appetite. Constipation is relieved. The body becomes light. Those who suffer from a shortening of the legs due to a fracture of the hip or thigh bone or bones of the leg will be benefited by this Asan. The trunk muscles are contracted and relaxed and stretched. The spine is bent laterally on both sides and the muscles are fully stretched. This Asan keeps the spine very elastic.

17. SAVASAN

"Sava" means 'dead body.' When one performs this Asan it gives the appearance of a dead body. So it is named Savasan. This is a closing pose. You should do this after doing all the other exercises.

Technique

Spread a soft blanket and lie supine (on the back). Keep the hands on the ground by the sides. Let the legs be straight. Keep the heels together and the toes separated. Now relax all the muscles of the body. Breathe slowly and rhythmically. Give up planning and scheming. Keep your eyes closed. Relax all the muscles, the nerves and the organs. Start the relaxation process from the toes upwards. Then proceed to the calf muscles, gastronemius, soleus and plantaris muscles, muscles of the neck, face, etc. Decide on a system. See that the abdominal organs, the heart, chest and the brain are also relaxed. Do not sleep. In this pose you will enjoy perfect peace, ease, comfort and relaxation.

Benefits

The pleasant and exhilarating feeling can only be realised by those who can successfully do this Asan. Words cannot adequately describe the peace which the practitioner enjoys. Every one of you should enjoy it. If you are tired from hard work, perform this Asan for 5 minutes. You will be fit again to continue your hard work with the same old vigour. This is a blessing for all hard workers.

18. UDDIYANA BANDHA

Empty the lungs by strong and forcible expiration. Now contract and forcibly draw up the intestines and also the navel towards the back, so that the abdomen rests against the back of the body high up in the thoracic cavity. He who practises this Bandha constantly conquers death and becomes young. This helps a lot in keeping up Brahmacharya. Uddiyana Bandha is practised during Rechak and at the end of Rechak (exhalation). Uddiyana can be done in a sitting or a standing posture. When you practise this in the standing posture, place your hands on the thighs. Keep the legs apart and bend your trunk slightly.

Uddiyana Bandha imparts good health, strength, vigour and vitality to the practitioner. When it is combined with Nauli Kriya which consists in churning the abdomen, it serves as a powerful gastro-intestinal tonic. Uddiyana Bandha and Nauli Kriya are two potent weapons of the Yogi for combating against constipation, weak peristalsis of the intestines and the gastro-intestinal disorders of the alimentary system.

19. NAULI KRIYA

Nauli Kriya is intended for regenerating, invigorating and stimulating the abdominal viscera and the gastro-intestinal or alimentary system. For the practice of Nauli, you should know Uddiyana Bandha well. Uddiyana Bandha can be done even in a sitting posture; but Nauli should be done only while standing.

Expire forcibly through the mouth and so keep the lungs completely empty. Contract and forcibly draw the abdominal muscles towards the back. This is Uddiyana Bandha.

For practising Nauli, stand up. Keep the right leg a foot apart from the left leg. Rest your hands on the thighs.

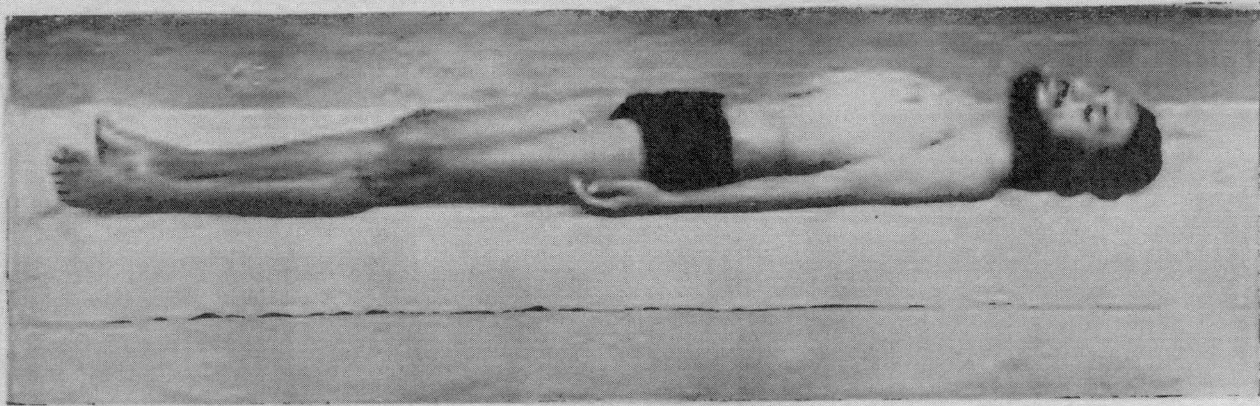

SAVASAN

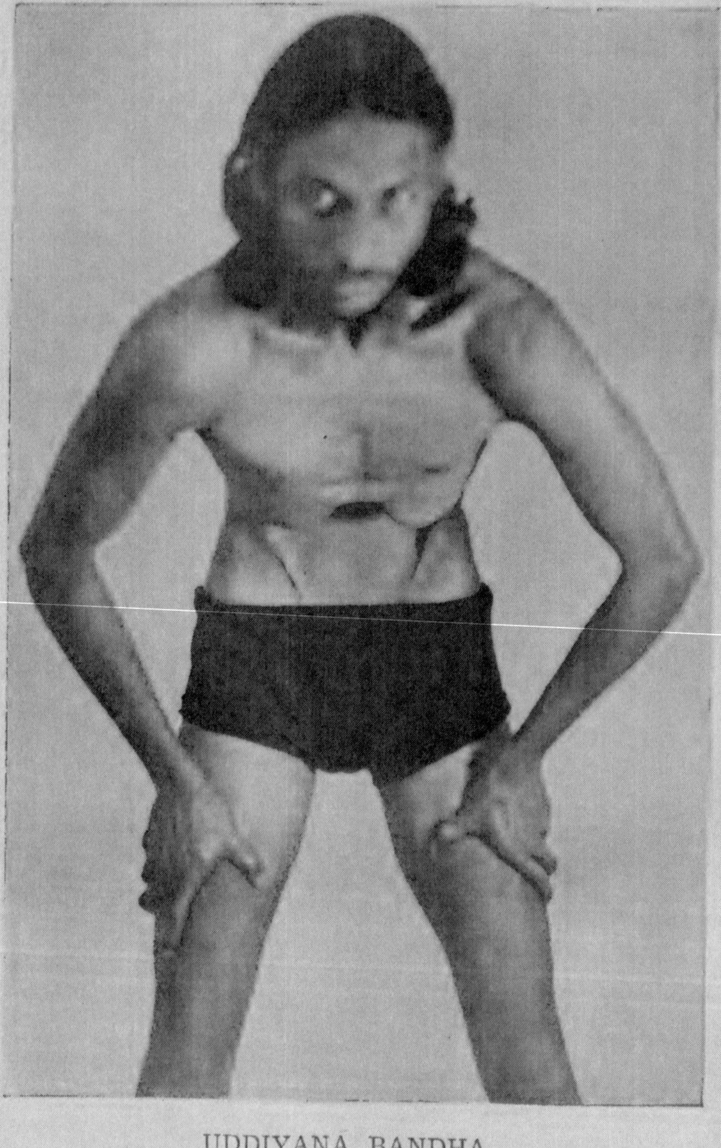

UDDIYANA BANDHA

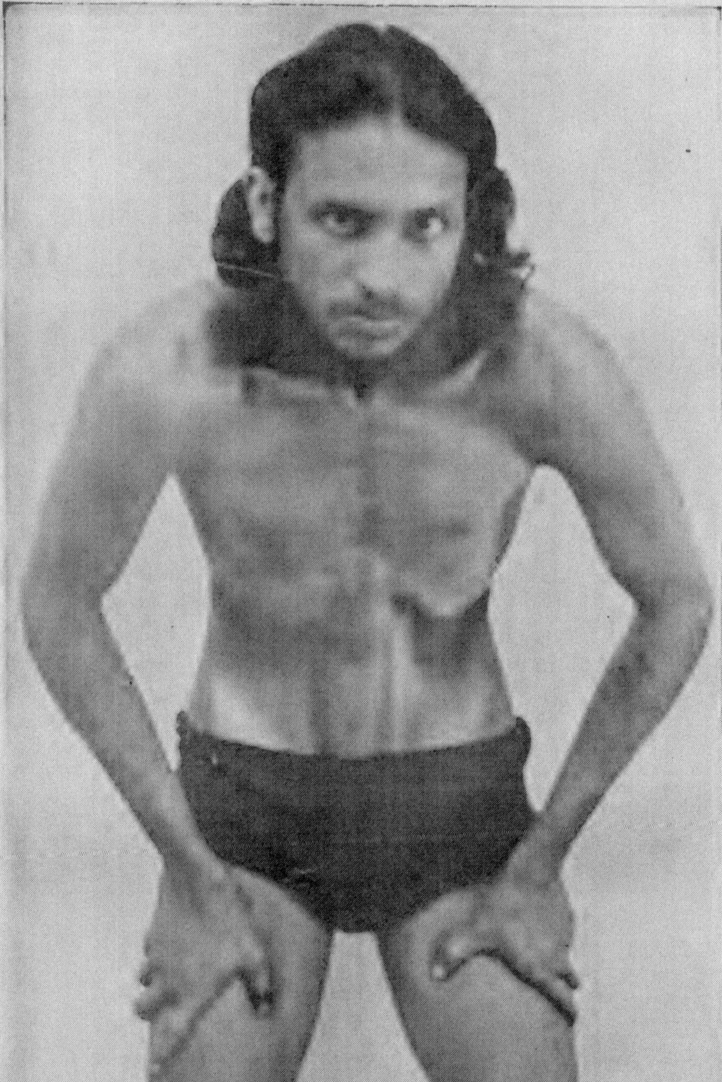

NAULI

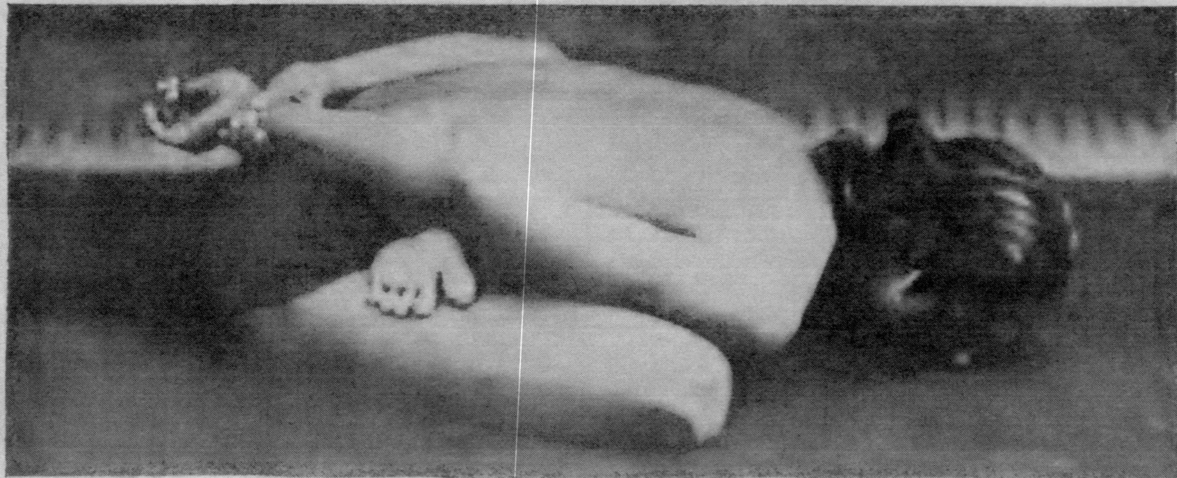

YOGA MUDRA

Slightly bend forward. Then do Uddiyana Bandha. Now allow the centre of the abdomen to be free by contracting the left and right side of the abdomen. You will have all the muscles in the centre in a vertical line. This is Madhyama Nauli.

Contract the right side of the abdomen and allow the left side to be free. You will have all the muscles on the left side only. This is Vama Nauli. Again contract the left side muscles and allow the right side to be free. This is Dakshina Nauli. By carrying out such graduated exercises you will understand how to contract the muscles of the central, left and right side of the abdominal muscles. You will also notice how they move from side to side. In this stage you will see the abdominal muscles only in the central, the right or on the left side.

Keep the muscles in the centre. Slowly bring them to the right side and then to the left side in a circular way. Do this several times from right to left and then do it in a reverse way from the left to the right side. When you advance, you may do these more quickly. This last stage of Nauli will appear like 'churning' when the abdominal muscles are isolated and rotated from side to side.

When Nauli is demonstrated by advanced students, the onlookers will be extremely surprised to see the movements of the abdominal muscles. They will feel as if an engine were working in the abdominal factory. Those who have a tender body, can very easily learn and perform this Kriya in a beautiful and efficient manner.

Nauli Kriya eradicates chronic constipation, dyspepsia and all other diseases of the gastro-intestinal system. The liver and pancreas are toned up. The kidneys and the other organs of the abdomen are also made to function properly.

20. YOGA MUDRA

Sit on a blanket. Form a foot-lock (Padmasan) by placing the right foot over the left thigh and the left foot over the right thigh. Slowly bend forward and touch the ground with the forehead. Take your hands to the back and catch hold of the right hand at the wrist by the left hand. As you bend down, exhale slowly. Remain in this pose for 10 seconds and then assume the original sitting posture and inhale slowly. Repeat the Mudra six times. This is very useful for rousing the Kundalini Shakti. This pose removes all kinds of disorders of the abdominal viscera.

21. SPECIAL INSTRUCTIONS

1. Get up at 4 a.m. Answer the calls of nature. Wash your face. Then practise your Asans, Pranayam exercises and meditation. This order is beneficial. If you are not in the habit of answering the calls of nature in the early morning, you should practise the Asans before answering the calls. It is advisable that Yogic students should practise all Asans after evacuating the bowels. If you are in the habit of defecating in the afternoon or evenings only, you should change this habit. You must be able to get one clear motion in the early morning as soon as you get up from bed. You can break any old habit and establish a healthy, new habit in course of time. Drink some cold or lukewarm water at night and in the early morning also as soon as you get up from bed. Regulate and adjust the diet also.

2. Wear a Longotee or Kowpeen or suspensory bandage when you practise Asans. You can have a banian on the body.

3. Do not wear spectacles when you do Asans. They may be broken and may injure your eyes.

4. Those who practise Sirshasan and other exercises for a long time, should take a little light food or a cup of milk after finishing the course.

5. Be regular in the practice of Asans. Those who practise by fits and starts will not derive much benefit from them.

6. If one takes to Yogic practices without observing moderation in diet he will not obtain the full benefits of these exercises.

7. The superstructure of a building will fall down in no time if the foundation is not properly laid. Even so a Yogic

student cannot proceed successfully in the higher courses if he has not gained mastery in Asans.

8. Regularity in practice is very necessary if one wants to realise the maximum benefits of Asans and Pranayams. Generally people practise for two months in the beginning with great interest and enthusiasm and then suddenly leave off the practice. This is a sad mistake. Practise the Asans and Pranayams regularly for a long time and realise the marvellous benefits derivable from them.

9. Physical exercises draw the Prana out. Asans send the Prana in. Asans distribute Prana quite evenly throughout the body and its different systems. Asans are not only physical but also spiritual as they awaken the Kundalini Shakti. A particular Asan removes a particular disease. Asans are preventives also.

10. Asans are not mere physical exercises. They are something more than that. They have a spiritual basis. They help much in controlling the senses, the mind and the body. The body, the nerves and the muscles are purified.

11. Ladies also should practise Asans. They will have healthy and strong children. If mothers are healthy and strong, the children also will be healthy and strong. Regeneration of the ladies means the regeneration of the whole world. If ladies practise a course of Asans systematically with interest and attention, they will have wonderful health and vitality. There is no doubt about this.

12. In the beginning you will not be able to perform some of the poses perfectly. Regular practice for some days will bring perfection. Patience and perseverance, earnestness and sincerity are needed.

13. Commonsense should be used throughout your practice. If one kind of food is not agreeable to your system, change the diet. If a particular Asan is not suitable to you select some other Asan. This is Yukti.

14. If you cannot perform a particular Asan quite satisfactorily, do not lose heart. Where there is a will there is

a way. Try, try and try again. Continual practice will make you perfect ultimately.

15. If you are careful about your diet, Asans and meditation, you will have fine, lustrous eyes, a fair and clear complexion and peace of mind. Yoga ensures beauty, health, strength and long life to its practitioners.

16. Brahmacharya is very very important. Evil thoughts are the beginning of adultery. Even the idea of lust must not enter the mind. You can realise the maximum benefits of Asans and Pranayams if you observe Brahmacharya strictly.

17. Do not wear heavy clothes. Light clothing permits the air to come into free contact with the skin. The latter is the most important eliminative agent in the whole bodily system. If its normal functions are weakened by the use of too much clothing poisons will accumulate.

18. Abandon devitalising habits. Any habit which tends to lower the tone of the bodily system will bring on various sorts of diseases. Anything which tends to lower the vitality lowers the system's power of elimination. The use of alcoholic liquors, tobacco, cocaine, opium, gunja or canabis indica, dissipations and excess of any kind should be given up entirely.

19. Asans should be practised both in the early morning and the evening. They should not be done immediately after meals as the bodily energy is freely utilised in assisting digestion. They may be practised five hours after taking food in the evening. Asans should be practised in a well-ventilated room, on an open terrace, on a river bank, the sea-shore or in the garden.

20. Immediately after performing Asans and Pranayams, no physical exercises should be done, because all the Asans tone up the internal organs and tissues. So the blood has to be supplied freely to these systems and tissues. But physical exercise is intended to tone up only the muscles, so the blood will be drawn to them only. The circulation

of blood in this case is completely opposite, and the benefits of Asans will be nullified. After doing Asans, take rest for a few minutes and then begin your physical exercises.

21. No Samadhi or super-conscious state is possible without awakening first the Kundalini Shakti. Kundalini can be awakened in various ways, viz., the practice of Asans, Mudras, Bandhas, Pranayams, devotion, grace of a Guru, Japa, strong analytic will and Vichara Shakti. Those who try to awaken the Kundalini should have perfect purity of thought, word and deed. They should have mental and physical Brahmacharya. Then only can they enjoy the benefits of Samadhi. You will be freed from the wheel of Samsara (wheel of births and deaths) and will attain Immortal Sat-chit-ananda state eventually.

CHAPTER II

PRANAYAM

1. PRANA AND PRANAYAM

Prana is the universal principle of energy or force. It is the vital force. It is all-pervading. It may be either in a static or dynamic state. It is found in all forms from the highest to the lowest, from the ant to the elephant, from the unicellular amoeba to a man, from the elementary forms of plant life to the developed forms of animal life. It is Prana that shines in your eyes. It is through the power of Prana that the ear hears, the eyes see, the skin feels, the tongue tastes, the nose smells, the brain and the intellect do their functions. The smile in a young lady, the melody in the music, the power in the emphatic words of an orator, the charm in the speech of one's beloved are all due to Prana. Fire burns through pranas. Wind blows through Prana. River flows through Prana. The aeroplane moves in the air through Prana. The steam engine works through Prana. Trains and motor cars move through Prana. Radio waves travel through Prana. Prana is electron. Prana is force. Prana is magnetism. Prana is electricity. It is Prana that pumps the blood from the heart into the arteries of blood-vessels. It is Prana that is responsible for the processes of digestion, excretion, and secretion.

Prana is expended by thinking, willing, acting, moving, talking, writing, etc. A healthy, strong man has abundance of Prana or nerve-force or vitality. The Prana is supplied by food, water, air, solar energy, etc. The supply of Prana is taken up by the nervous system. The Prana is absorbed by breathing. The excess of Prana is stored in the brain and nerve centres. When the seminal energy sublimates, or transforms, it supplies abundance of Prana to the system. It is stored up in the brain in the form of Ojas. Ojas is nothing but Prana.

The Yogi stores abundance of Prana by a regular practice of Pranayam just as a storage battery can be made to store electricity. That Yogi who has stored up a large supply of Prana radiates strength and vitality all round. He is a mighty power-house. Those who come in close contact with him imbibe Prana from him, and get strength, vigour, vitality and exhilaration of spirits. Just as water flows from one vessel to another, Prana actually flows like a steady current from a developed Yogi towards weak persons. This can be actually seen by the Yogi who has developed his inner Yogic vision.

Pranayam is the control of the Prana and the vital forces of the body. It is regulation of the breath. This is a most important step. The aim of Pranayam is the control of Prana. Pranayam begins with the regulation of the breath for having control over the life-currents through the control of breath. Breath is the external manifestation of the gross Prana. A correct habit of breathing must be established by the regular practice of Pranayam. In ordinary worldly persons the breathing is irregular.

If you can control the Prana you can completely control all the forces of the universe, mental and physical. The Yogi can also control the omnipresent manifesting power out of which all energies take their origin, whether magnetism, electricity, gravitation, cohesion, nerve-currents, vital forces or thought vibrations; in fact the total forces of the universe—physical and mental.

If one controls breath or Prana, the mind is also controlled. He who has controlled his mind has also controlled his breath. If one is suspended, the other is also suspended. If the mind and the Prana are both controlled one gets liberation from the round of births and deaths and attains immortality. There is an intimate connection between the mind, Prana and semen. If one controls the seminal energy, the mind and Prana are also controlled. He who has controlled his seminal force has also controlled his Prana and mind.

When you wish to hear a faint sound, the breath gets automatically suspended for a short time. The cooly who carries heavy bags of rice at the railway station instinctively fills his lungs with air and practises unconscious retention of the air (Pranayam) till the bag is lifted on to his back. He who crosses a small rivulet by jumping, he who practises long jump and high jump and various exercises with the parallel bars practises retention of breath instinctively. This retention of breath augments his vitality, strength. It provides abundance of energy immediately.

Just as a goldsmith removes impurities from gold by heating it in a hot furnace and by blowing strongly through a blow-pipe, so also the Yogic student removes the impurities of the body and the indriyas by blowing his lungs, i.e., by practising Pranayam.

The chief aim of Pranayam is to unite the Prana with the Apana and take the united Prana-apana slowly upwards to the head. The effect or fruit of Pranayam is awakening of the sleeping Kundalini.

Pranayam though it concerns the breath only, gives good exercise also to the various internal organs and the whole body. Pranayam removes all sorts of diseases, improves health, energises digestion, invigorates the nerves, removes passion and awakens Kundalini Shakti. It bestows good health and a steady mind. A Pranayam practitioner can stop his breath. People can break stones on his chest. He does not feel anything because he has controlled his Prana. A Pranayam practitioner will have a light body free from diseases, a very fair complexion, a sweet melodious voice, and a pleasant smell from his body.

He who practises Pranayam will have good appetite, cheerfulness, a handsome figure, great strength, courage, enthusiasm, a high standard of health, vigour and vitality and good concentration of the mind. This Pranayam is quite suitable for people in the West and East, men and women.

A Yogi measures the span of his life not by the number of years but by the number of breaths. You take in a certain amount of energy or Prana from the atmosphere along with each breath. Vital capacity is the capacity of a man to inhale the largest quantity of air after the deepest possible exhalation. A man takes fifteen breaths in a minute. So the total number of breaths amounts to 21,600 per day.

The room in which you practise Pranayam must not be damp or ill-ventilated. It must be dry and airy. You may practise by the side of a river or lake, in the corner of a garden in the open air, when there is no chill or draught of cold air or on the top or foot of a hill. The practice of Pranayam should be performed daily with the mind firmly fixed on Truth. Then the Chitta is absorbed in the Sushumna. Consequently the Prana becomes steady. It does not fluctuate. Pranayam requires deep concentration and attention.

There should be no strain at any stage in the practice of Pranayam. You should experience joy and pleasure in doing the same. You should not feel any undue strain. Always inhale and exhale very very slowly. Do not make the least sound. Whenever you feel uneasy, depressed, or dejected, practise Pranayam.

The practice of Kumbhak (retention) in Pranayam produces heat and thereby the Kundalini Shakti is awakened and passes upwards along the Sushumna Nadi. Kumbhak increases the period of life also. Mild Kumbhak during the practice of Asans augments the efficacy of Asans and gives increased power and vitality. During the practice of Pranayam repeat your Ishta Mantra (Japa). That will be pure Yoga.

As there is always some drowsiness when one gets up from bed, it is advisable to do a few Pranayams, 10 to 20 mild Kumbhak just to drive off drowsiness and to make you fit for meditation. The mind gets one-pointed after the practice of Pranayam.

2. SUKH PURVAK

(Easy Comfortable Pranayam)

Sit in the Padmasan or Siddhasan pose in your meditation room. Close the right nostril with the right thumb. Draw in the air very slowly through the left nostril. Then close the left nostril also with the little and ring fingers of the right hand. Retain the air as long as you can comfortably keep. Then exhale very very slowly through the right nostril after removing the thumb.

Then draw in the air through the right nostril. Retain the air as before and exhale it very very slowly through the left nostril after removing the little and ring fingers. All these six processes constitute one Pranayam. Do 5 Pranayams to start with and increase the number gradually. You can do 20 Pranayams at a sitting.

Have a Bhav (mental attitude) that all the Deivi Sampat (Divine qualities) such as mercy, love, forgiveness, santi, joy, etc., are entering into your system along with the inspired air and that all the Asura Sampat (devilish qualities) such as lust, anger, greed, etc., are being thrown out along with the expired air. Repeat OM mentally during Purak (inhalation), Kumbhak (retention) and Rechak (exhalation).

This Pranayam removes all diseases, purifies the Nadis, steadies the mind in concentration, improves digestion, increases the digestive fire and the appetite, helps to maintain Brahmacharya and awakens the Kundalini Shakti. Purification of Nadis will set in rapidly.

For Purak, Kumbhak and Rechak, the ratio is 1 : 4 : 2. If you inhale for 4 seconds, retain the air for 16 seconds and then exhale for 8 seconds. You can gradually increase these to 16, 64 and 32 seconds respectively.

3. UJJAYI

Adopt the Padmasan or the Siddhasan pose. Close the mouth. Inhale slowly through both the nostrils in a smooth uniform manner till the breath seems to fill the space between the throat and the heart. Retain the breath as long as you can comfortably and then exhale through the left nostril by closing the right nostril with your right thumb. Expand the chest when you exhale. During inhalation a peculiar sound is produced owing to the partial closing of the glottis. The sound produced during inhalation should be of a mild and uniform pitch. It should be continuous also. This Pranayam can be practised even while walking or standing. Instead of exhaling through the left nostril, you can exhale slowly through both nostrils.

This Pranayam removes the heat in the head. The gastric fire is increased. It removes phlegm from the throat. Asthma, consumption and all sorts of pulmonary diseases are cured. Everything is accomplished by Ujjayi. The practitioner is never attacked by diseases of phlegm, nerves, dyspepsia, dysentery, enlarged spleen, consumption, cough, or fever. Perform Ujjayi to destroy decay and prevent death.

4. SITALI

Protrude the tongue a little away from the lips. Fold the tongue like a tube, lengthwise. Draw in the air through the mouth with the hissing sound *SI*. Retain the breath as long as you can with comfort. Then exhale slowly through both the nostrils. Practise this 6 times. You can do this even while standing or walking.

This Pranayam purifies the blood. It quenches thirst and appeases hunger. It destroys Gulma (chronic dyspepsia), inflammation of various chronic diseases, fever, consumption, indigestion, bilious disorders, etc. You will find this extremely useful in summer.

5. BHASTRIKA

In Sanskrit "Bhastrika" means bellows. Rapid succession of forcible expulsions is a characteristic feature of Bhastrika. Just as a blacksmith blows his bellows rapidly, so also you will have to move your breath rapidly.

Sit in Padmasan. Keep the body, neck and head erect. Close the mouth. Now inhale and exhale quickly ten times like the bellows of a blacksmith. Constantly dilate and contract the chest. Forcibly and quickly inhale and exhale ten times and then make a deep inhalation through both the nostrils. Retain the breath as long as you can do with comfort and then exhale completely. This is one round of Bhastrika. You can do this 4 times. After some practice, you can gradually increase the number of expulsions to 20. You can do 10 rounds in a sitting. You will not feel any fatigue, if you take a little rest after each round. Take a few normal breaths after each round. Then you will be fresh for the next round.

The number of expulsions for each round is determined by the strength and capacity of the practitioner. You must not go to extremes. Practise regularly every day and gradually increase the number of rounds.

There is another variety of Bhastrika wherein only one nostril is used for breathing purposes.

Bhastrika is a powerful exercise. It relieves inflammation of the throat, increases the gastric fire, destroys phlegm, removes diseases of the nose and chest and cures asthma and consumption. It removes all diseases which arise from an excess of wind, bile and phlegm. It gives warmth to the body. It purifies the Nadis considerably. It is the most beneficial of all Kumbhaks. It awakens Kundalini Shakti quickly. For health and strength, practise Bhastrika.

CHAPTER III

RELAXATION

1. SCIENCE OF RELAXATION

Life has become very complex in these days. The struggle for existence is very acute and keen. There is very unhealthy competition in every walk of life. The bread problem has become very difficult. There is unemployment everywhere. Brilliant young men with extraordinary qualifications and recommendations alone get a job in these days. Therefore a great deal of continuous mental and physical strain is imposed on modern humanity by its deadening daily work and unhealthy mode of life.

Action produces movement; movements cause habits. Man has acquired many artificial habits. He has allowed nature's original habits to lapse. He has brought tension in many muscles and nerves through incorrect habit-positions. He has forgotten the first principles of relaxation. He will have to learn lessons from the cat, dog and the infant in the Science of Relaxation.

If you practise relaxation no energy will be wasted. You will be very active and energetic. During relaxation the muscles and nerves are at rest. The Prana or energy is stored up and conserved. The vast majority of persons who have no comprehensive understanding of this beautiful science of relaxation simply waste their energies by creating unnecessary movements of muscles and by putting the muscles and nerves under great strain.

Some persons shake their legs unnecessarily while sitting. Some play Mridang or Tabla (drum) with their fingers on the table when their minds are idle or vacant. Some whistle. Some shake their heads. Some tap their chests or abdomen with their fingers. Energy is thus dissipated through unnecessary movements of the different parts of the body on account of lack of knowledge of the elementary principles of the science of relaxation.

Do not mistake laziness for relaxation. The lazy man is inactive. He has no inclination for work. He is full of lethargy and inertia. He is dull. Whereas a man who practises relaxation takes only rest. He has vigour, strength, vitality and endurance. He never allows even a small amount of energy to trickle away. He accomplishes wonderful work gracefully in a minimum amount of time.

When you wish to contract a muscle in order to perform an action an impulse is transmitted from the brain through the nerve to the muscle. Energy or Prana travels through the motor nerves, reaches the muscle and causes it to draw its ends together. When the muscle contracts it pulls up the limb which you wish to move. Now you can perform the action with ease. First there is thought. Thought takes form in action through contraction of muscles.

Suppose you wish to lift up a chair. The desire creates an impulse in the brain. The impulse is transmitted to the muscles of the arms from the brain through the motor nerves. A current of Prana or energy is transmitted along the nerves from the brain. The muscles contract and you perform the action of lifting up the chair. Similarly all other actions, conscious or unconscious, are performed by you. If the muscles are overworked more energy is spent and you feel fatigue. There is much wear and tear in the muscles through overwork, strain and tension on account of heavy expenditure of Prana or energy.

When you perform an action consciously a message is given to the mind and the mind immediately obeys by sending a current of energy to the desired part. An unconscious act is done instinctively or mechanically. The mind does not wait for orders. When the scorpion stings your finger, the finger is at once withdrawn. You do not argue here. This is an instinctive or mechanical movement.

A man of easily irritable nature cannot enjoy peace of mind. His brain, nerves and muscles are always under high tension. He is wasting every minute abundant muscular and nerve energy and brain-power. He is a very weak man though he may be endowed with physical strength, because he loses his balance of mind very easily. If you really want to enjoy unruffled peace and abiding joy you must try to possess a calm, controlled and balanced mind by eradicating worry, anxieties, fear, anger impulses and repressing impulses.

You do not gain anything by worrying yourself unnecessarily and manifesting anger for nothing at all. Anger belongs to a brutal nature. Anger does positive injury to the brain, the blood and the nerves. You are not profited a bit by exhibiting anger. By repeating an action, a habit is formed in the mind. If you worry yourself frequently, a worrying habit is developed. Your vitality and energy are simply drained by worry, anger and fear. Why should you be afraid of anything at all, when everything is nothing but your own self? Fear, anger and worry are the products of ignorance. The muscles and nerves of a victim of anger and worry are always under contraction and high tension.

The action of one set of muscles can be checked by the operation of another set of muscles. One impulse may try to put one set of muscles in motion and by sending another repressive impulse through another set of muscles you can counteract the action of the first set of muscles. If a man abuses you, you may jump at once to beat him. An impulse has already put one set of muscles in motion. You may check the impulse through discrimination and reflection : "I do not gain anything by beating him. He is an ignorant man. He does not know how to behave. Let me forgive him now." A repressive impulse will check at once the operation of the first set of muscles by another set of muscles. Raising of impulses and counter-impulses or repressing impulses cause high tension in nerves, muscles and brain. A large number of people are slaves of impulses; hence they do not enjoy peace of mind. They are tossed hither and thither.

The science of relaxation is an exact science. It can be learnt very easily. Relaxation of the muscles is as important as contraction of the muscles. I lay great emphasis on the relaxation of the mind, the nerves and the muscles.

Relaxation is of two kinds, viz., Mental Relaxation and Physical Relaxation. There is another classification. If you relax certain muscles of certain parts only, it is partial relaxation. If you relax all the muscles of the whole body, it is complete relaxation.

2. PHYSICAL RELAXATION

EXERCISE NO. 1

You must know how to relax all the muscles of your body after you have finished your daily course of exercises. The practice of relaxing the muscles of the body will bring rest to the body and the mind also. The tension of the muscles of the body will be relieved. People who know the science of relaxation do not waste any energy. They can meditate well.

After finishing your exercises and Asans, lie down flat on your back. Keep the hands on the sides quite relaxed. Keep them quite loose. You may practise Savasan or Murdhasan. Relax all the muscles from head to foot. Roll the mind over the body from top to toe. You may find that certain muscles are not completely relaxed. Relax them also.

Roll on to one side and then relax as thoroughly as you can. Do not strain any muscles. Relax completely. Roll on to the other side and then relax again. This is done naturally by all during sleep. There are various exercises for relaxation for the particular muscles of the different parts of the body. You can relax the head, the shoulder, the arms, the forearms, the wrist, fingers, thighs, legs, ankles, toes, knees, elbows, the waist, etc. Yogis and Phailwans know the science of relaxation thoroughly. When you practise these various exercises in relaxation, you must bear in your mind a picture of calmness and strength.

If you like you can practise relaxation by lying in an easy chair after finishing your Asans or exercises. Those who know relaxation can take a short nap of ten minutes or so at any time they like. Busy people, doctors and lawyers should know the science of relaxation. They can relax the mind also and take rest in the waiting rooms of railway stations and bar rooms as well. They will thus be quite fit for further activity in the courts or the dispensary. Relaxation refreshes a man completely.

Students, journalists, busy lawyers, doctors and business men should know the science of mental relaxation. They should practise it daily. Those who do not possess a knowledge of this science of internal and external relaxation waste their physical and mental energy considerably. Those who practise relaxation can conserve their physical and mental energy and utilise it to their best advantage. Yogis know this science well. They are perfect masters of this useful science. Those who practise relaxation will never experience fatigue. They can close their eyes for a few minutes even while standing and so prepare themselves for further work. Energy flows in their nerves when they relax just as water flows when the tap is turned open.

EXERCISE NO. II (FOR WOMEN)

The woman who can never relax, never take a real rest, will not retain beauty. Her face will show signs of the fatigue her body is undergoing. Her body will lack poise. By being in a continual state of nervous tension (as many women are) she will grow old before her time, lose her looks, find that the tension has sapped all her strength away.

Once in the morning and once in the afternoon, relax completely for ten minutes at least. No matter how urgent the task, stick to this rule. Sit on a very comfortable chair, or lie flat on a mattress; prop up the legs about eighteen inches from the ground with a stiff cushion under the knees, and let every muscle go 'flop.' A cushion under the head, if lying on the mattress, will relax the neck muscles. Close the eyes. Make the mind blank.

The idea of propping up the legs is to make the spine lie flat and to cool the feet by letting the blood run away from them. When resting in a chair, prop up the legs and relax every muscle. It will not come easily at first, but it can be turned into a habit.

There are many jobs which can be done in a sitting position—darning, mending and sewing, machine work. Be careful to sit correctly in order to avoid fatigue. Only a few women are aware of the fact that a faulty position may enlarge the hips. Never sit on the edge of a chair. Place the body well back and have a firm cushion to support the lower part of the back. Another thing to remember is to choose a chair of the correct height. Do not cross the legs. Sit with the knees and feet close together and firmly planted on the floor or on a stool.

Fatigue can be avoided at other tasks by adopting a correct standing posture. When a job necessitates your being on the feet for a long time, keep the knees and heels close together. This makes a pillar on which the body can rest. The weight of the body is not thrown on one leg or the other, but is distributed evenly on both.

3. MENTAL RELAXATION

EXERCISE NO. I

Just as you relax your muscles after having finished your Asans and physical exercises, so also you will have to relax the mind and rest it after concentration and meditation after the practice of memory training and will-culture. Relaxation of the muscles brings repose to the mind. Relaxation of the mind brings rest to the body as well. The body and mind are intimately connected. The body is a mould prepared by the mind for its enjoyment.

The mind gathers experiences through the body and works in conjunction with the Prana, senses and body. The mind has influence over the body. If you are cheerful the body also will be healthy and strong. When you are feeling depressed, the body cannot work. Conversely the body has some influence over the mind. If the body is healthy and strong, the mind will also be happy, cheerful and strong. If there is a stomachache, the mind cannot work. Thought takes form in action and action reacts on the mind. The mind acts on the body and the body reacts on the mind.

Removal of tension in the muscles brings repose and calmness to the mind.

By relaxation you give rest to the mind, tired nerves and the overworked muscles. You will get immense peace of mind, strength and vigour. When you practise relaxation of either body or mind, the brain should not be occupied with various sorts of loose extraneous thoughts. Anger, disappointment, failure, indisposition, misery, sorrow, quarrels cause internal mental strain. The practice of relaxation of mind will remove internal mental strain and will fill the mind with new mental energy and will make you cheerful and happy.

Mental poise and calmness may be brought about by the eradication of worry and anger. Fear really underlies both worry and anger. Nothing is gained by worry and anger, but on the contrary much energy is wasted by these two kinds of lower emotions. Be careful and thoughtful. All unnecessary worries should be avoided. Expel from you all fear, worry and anger. Think of courage, joy, bliss, peace and cheerfulness. Sit for fifteen minutes in a relaxed state and an easy comfortable position. You can lie on an easy chair. Close your eyes. Withdraw the mind from outside objects. Still the mind. Silence the bubbling thoughts.

EXERCISE NO. II

Close the eyes. Think of anything that is pleasant. This will relax the mind in a wonderful manner. Think of the mighty Himalayas, the sacred Ganges, and striking scenery in Kashmir, the Taj Mahal, the Victoria Memorial in Calcutta, a lovely sunset, the vast expanse of ocean or the infinite blue sky. Imagine that the whole world and your body are floating like a straw in this vast ocean of spirit. Feel that you are in touch with the Supreme Being. Feel that the life of the whole world is pulsating, vibrating and throbbing through you. Feel that Lord Hiranyagarbha, the ocean of life, is gently rocking you on His vast bosom. Then open your eyes. You will experience immense mental peace, mental vigour and mental strength. Practise and feel this.

APPENDIX

1. YOGIC ALPHABET

Asans make you strong and healthy and eradicate many diseases.

Bhastrika Pranayama develops the lungs and destroys the germs of tuberculosis and augments lung-power and lung-capacity.

Constipation is removed by the practice of Bhujang, Salabh and Dhanur Asans.

Dhanurasan is a combination of Bhujang and Salabh Asans.

Eating in moderation, simple living and high thinking help the Yogic student to attain his goal quickly.

Fasting eliminates poison, purifies the whole bodily system and invigorates the cells.

Garbhasan augments the digestive power, increases the appetite and removes many intestinal diseases.

Halasan makes the spine very elastic and very supple.

Indriyas should be controlled by the practice of Pratyahara and Dama.

Japa of OM or Hari OM should go hand in hand with Asan and Pranayama.

Kumbhak helps to attain longevity and awaken the Kundalini.

Lolasan strengthens the muscles of the arms and forearms.

Mind can be controlled by Vairagya, Abhyasa, Sat Sang, Vichara, eradication of Vasanas, destruction of egoism, Pranayama, meditation and cultivation of virtues such as mercy, complacency, self-denial, santi and Santosh.

Nadi Suddhi can be obtained by the practice of Pranayama.

Oordhva Padmasan checks wet-dreams, transmutes the sexual energy into Ojas.

Paschimottanasan removes fat, increases the gastric fire and cures diseases of the stomach.

Quetta Earthquake is nothing when compared to the agitation caused in the mind by the turbulent senses.

Regularity in the practice of Asan and Pranayama is an indispensable requisite for quick and solid progress.

Sirshasan is King of All Asans. It transmutes seminal energy into Ojas, develops memory and intellectual capacity and cures a host of ailments.

Tratak helps concentration of the mind and removes diseases of the eyes.

Uddiyana Bandha imparts beautiful health, strength, vigour, and vitality and removes the disorders of the alimentary system.

Vajrasan removes drowsiness, strengthens the spine, helps digestion and is very useful for meditation.

Winter is the best time for a rigorous practice of Yoga.

Xerostomia or abnormal dryness of the mouth can be removed by the practice of Sitali and Sitakari Pranayama.

Yoga Mudra cures the disorders of the abdomen and awakens the Kundalini.

Zerosis is a disease of the eye caused by a deficiency of vitamin 'A'. This is removed by the practice of mild Tratak and Sirshasan.

2. THE GOAL OF LIFE

In the whirlpool of fleeting sensual pleasures you have forgotten the purpose of life and the goal. You live more for the body than for the soul. In your pursuit after the phantom shows of worldly vanities, you have annihilated the spiritual instincts and longings of the soul. What a sad state! Mysterious is Maya! Mysterious is Moha! Open your eyes now. Wake up from the long slumber of ignorance. Realise the ultimate Reality and enjoy the eternal Bliss.

Spiritual wealth is the real inexhaustible wealth. Spiritual knowledge is the real knowledge. Spiritual life is the real life. Aspire. Know thy Self and be free. Regain the lost Divine Glory. Meditate and realise the Immortal Atma, the indweller of your heart, the inner Ruler, the Self-existent, Self-contained, Self-luminous imperishable soul.

This is a world of diversity. Intellects are different. Faces are different. Religions are different. Sounds are different. Faiths are different. Colours are different. But one thing is common in all. Every one of us wants Nitya Sukha (eternal happiness), infinite Knowledge, Immortality, freedom and independence. These things can be obtained by a knowledge of the Self alone.

Everybody wants eternal happiness or happiness that is not mixed with sorrow and pain. Every human effort is to achieve this happiness. But he does not know the peace wherefrom he can get this supreme bliss. If you want to enjoy supreme bliss you will have to realise the Self, or get knowledge of Atma. The best means to acquire this knowledge is the enquiry of 'Who am I?' This enquiry has the potentiality of producing the quietness of mind which will enable it to wade through this ocean of Samsara. But this enquiry demands a subtle, sharp, pure intellect, bold understanding and gigantic will.

The goal of life is the attainment of Self-realisation or God-consciousness. There is one supreme undying intelligent principle or Essence or Atma or Brahman or the Supreme Self who dwells in the chambers of your heart. He exists in the past, present and future. He is existence Absolute, knowledge Absolute and bliss Absolute. Ignorant man vainly searches for his happiness in perishable external objects, that are conditioned by time, space and causation. He has no peace of mind. His desires are not gratified. He amasses wealth, begets children, gets titles, honours, name, fame and yet his mind is restless. He has no abiding joy and lasting happiness. He is still in want of something. He has no feeling of fullness. This feeling of fullness and eternal satisfaction can only be obtained by realising one's own Self through self-restraint, purity and meditation.

There is restlessness everywhere. Selfishness, greed, wrath, lust abound on all sides. Fights, skirmishes, petty quarrels are polluting the atmosphere and creating discord, disharmony and unrest. The bugle is blown and soldiers are marching to the battlefield to kill their enemies. One nation is waging war against another nation for acquiring more dominions and more power. Side by side the peace movement is working silently for bringing concord, harmony and peace, for eradicating the dire ignorance, the root-cause of all human sufferings and disseminating Divine Knowledge or Knowledge of the Self and infusing devotion into the hearts of the people. Mysterious is the universe ! Still more mysterious is the silent workings of the unseen God, who prompts Rajasic people on one side to wage war and the Sattwic people on the other side to start peace-centres for the dissemination of spiritual knowledge and for bringing peace to suffering humanity at large. Lord Jesus says: "Blessed are the peace-makers ! for they shall be called the children of God."

How long do you want to lead a life of duality, restlessness, discontentment and dissatisfaction? How long do you wish to lead a life of ignorance, bitterness, hatred and separation? How long do you wish to continue your selfish struggles? How long do you want to behold differences and distinctions? How long do you wish to keep your barrier between man and man?

Peace is not merely the absence of noise, tumult, strife or quarrels, controversies or disputes. It can hardly be acquired from external sources. It is not a condition of environment from which all undesirable elements are removed. If three Sadhus live in a solitary cave in the Himalayas, if they fight amongst themselves, if they harbour in their hearts jealousy, hatred and ill-will, they will pollute the most peaceful environment and the tranquil atmosphere of the place. In this state (of peace) there are no yesterdays and no tomorrows, no sunset and no dawns. There is eternal sunshine.

Peace, God, Atma, Brahman, Freedom, Immortality, Kaivalya, Nirvana, Moksha, Param-Dama, Paramananda, Prapthi are synonymous terms. Righteousness and peace kiss each other. Love and peace embrace each other. Peace and unity walk together with clasped hands. Desirelessness moves hand in hand with peace. There can be no peace without love of God.

The kingdom of peace is beyond all speech, thought and imagination. It can be reached only by patient spiritual practices. This peace is not an inert passive state. It is not a hypnotic trance. It is not a negative psychical condition. It is a positive state of the spiritual attainment. It is your centre, ideal and goal. It is the pivot of human life. It is soul's quest. It is perfect awareness. It is a magnanimous state in which the Yogi enjoys highest divine bliss and transcendental divine knowledge. The Yogi is in communion with the Supreme Soul or Paramatma. He becomes absolutely desireless and fearless, by drinking this divine nectar of peace.

Peace is your birthright. Peace is filling your beings within and without. Peace is in front of you, behind you, to the right, to the left, above and below. Peace is the only living reality. Names and forms are mere illusions. Realise this peace and be free. Wonderful is the power of peace that brings joy and eternal bliss.

Cross the wide ocean of strife by calming the mind through ceaseless meditation and reach the other shore of peace, fearlessness and immortality. Give up all selfish efforts and free yourself from the wild unrest of life.

Be still. Be in tune with the divine will. Let go all your worries. Cast out all cares and anxieties. Get deep down into the innermost recesses of your heart and plunge in the ocean of peace.

Live according to the Divine law of love or the golden rule. First endeavour to harmonise your own affairs. Establish first the kingdom of peace within your own heart. It is individual peace that paves the way towards universal Peace. The attainment of an inner calm is the greatest work you can do for humanity. A Yogi who has realised the peace that passeth understanding radiates peace to all the corners of the world. Those who come in contact with him are influenced by his sweet, soul-elevating harmonious vibrations. Hatred ceases in his presence.

It is useless to talk of the abolition of war while you are all full of petty jealousy and private hatred. Remove your discordant, inharmonious vibrations first. There will be no more war between nations then. Individuals go to constitute a nation. Lead an ideal life of peace. Kill ruthlessly all suspicion, prejudice of all sorts, envy, jealousy, selfishness, greed for power and possessions. Lead a simple life. Practise meditation daily and establish peace in your own heart. Then radiate it to your neighbours and all who come in contact with you. Disseminate it far and wide. Preach the gospel of peace to all men and women of the world.

If you annihilate selfishness, greed and egoism, Mother Nature will work for you. Co-operate with her, and she will carry your burden of life on her head. You can remain quite at ease. You will be free from care, worries, anxieties, responsibilities and fear. The individual will become one with cosmic will. Her aim and your aim will become one. Everything will become easy. Sadhana will go on by leaps and bounds. There will be no obstacles or impediments on your way. She will do everything for you. Whosoever surrenders his selfish aims and interests to the Will of the Lord will enjoy supreme peace and perennial bliss.

You will find in Gita: "The disciplined self, moving among sense-objects with senses free from attraction and repulsion mastered by the self, goeth to Peace. In that peace the extinction of all pains ariseth for him; for of him whose heart is peaceful the Reason soon attaineth equilibrium. There is no pure Reason for the non-harmonised, nor for the non-harmonised is there concentration; for him without concentration there is no peace, and for the unpeaceful how can there be happiness? Whoso forsaketh all desires and goeth onwards free from yearnings, selfishness and without egoism —he goeth to Peace" (II—64, 65, 66 and 67). "The man who is full of faith obtaineth wisdom, and he also who hath mastery over his senses: and having obtained wisdom he goeth swiftly to the supreme Peace." (Chap. IV—39.) "The Peace of the ETERNAL lies near to those who know themselves, who are disjoined from desire and anger, subdued in nature, of subdued thoughts." (V—26.)

Anger, greed, jealousy, hatred, are all enemies of peace. Develop goodwill, co-operation, mercy, compassion, non-resistance or non-retaliation to injuries done to you, forgiveness, contentment, nobility and cosmic love. Pray for him who has done you harm. Send thought-currents of peace and goodwill to him and the whole world at large when you sit for meditation.

You can find this Peace only in stillness. Sit silently in a quiet room from half-an-hour to one hour. Close your eyes. Relax the muscles and nerves. Concentrate on a point between the two eyebrows. Withdraw the senses and the mind from the external objects. Silence the surging emotions and bubbling thoughts. Forget the body and the world. Enter into the great calm or the secret Place of the Most High. You will find God who is Peace in the quietude of your inmost being. Have four sittings in winter and two in summer. Be regular in your practice. Regularity is of paramount importance. You can grow spiritually only if you are regular in your practice. If you yourself can enjoy peace, you can contribute peace to the world.

Attain to the peace that passeth understanding by silencing the bubbling thoughts and eradicating all desires, cravings or hankerings after worldly things. Reach the kingdom of inner stillness or domain of infinite peace through spiritual meditation. If you can still your mind you can still a tempest or a cyclone or the surging sea. Rest in the ocean of peace. Root your life in the Self within. Now you will be able to neutralise the dark forces of hatred, jealousy, disharmony, rupture and destruction.

Peace can be found only within. You certainly cannot find it in external objects. Wealth, women, children, property, palatial buildings cannot give you everlasting peace. Look within. Realise your oneness with the One Supreme—Intelligence and wisdom that dwell within the chambers of your heart. When you are established in the Highest Self within, you will not be shaken even by heavy sorrow, loss or failure, inharmonious or disagreeable vibrations. You will tide over all difficulties or crises of life easily and will come back with triumph in all life's experiences. Mysterious is this Peace! Marvellous is this Peace! Realise this Peace that passeth all understanding and be free. Float in this ocean of Peace and rejoice in the Peace of your own self. May this Peace guide you all. May this Peace be your ideal, centre and goal.

Peace be to the East. Peace be to the West. Peace be to the North. Peace be to the South. Peace be above. Peace be below. Peace be to all creatures of this universe.

3. CONTROL OF THOUGHT

The mind is like a wheel which revolves endlessly with tremendous velocity. It generates new thoughts with every revolution. This wheel is set in motion by the vibrations of psychic Prana or subtle Prana. The practice of Pranayama lessens the velocity of the mind, slows down the wheel gradually. Perfect control of Prana will bring the wheel to a standstill.

Alcohol, meat, rajasic foods, the cinema, novel-reading, obscene songs, obscene sights, obscene talks, evil company will make the wheel of mind revolve very rapidly; whereas fruits, sattwic food, the company of Mahatmas, study of religious books, solitude, Japa, kirtan, concentration, meditation, enquiry of "Who am I?" will slow down the wheel and eventually bring it to a standstill.

Identify yourself with the Immortal Self. Enquire "Who am I?" whenever bad thoughts arise in your mind. All the thoughts will gradually die.

The fewer the desires, the fewer the thoughts. Become absolutely desireless. The wheel of your mind will stop entirely. If you reduce your wants, if you do not try to fulfil your desires, if you try to eradicate your desires one by one your thoughts will diminish in frequency and length. The number of thoughts also per minute will decrease. Fewer the thoughts greater the peace. Remember this always. A wealthy man who speculates in a big city and who has a large number of thoughts has a restless mind, in spite of his comforts, whereas a Sadhu who lives in a cave on the Himalayas and who practises thought control is very happy in spite of his poverty.

The power of concentration will increase by lessening the number of thoughts. Certainly it is an uphill work to reduce the number of thoughts. In the beginning it will tax your ability very much. The task will be very unpleasant. But later on you will rejoice as you will get immense strength of mind and internal peace by reduction of thoughts. Armed with patience, perseverance, vigilance, fiery determination and iron will, you can crush the thoughts easily just as you crush a lemon or an orange, with ease. After crushing it will be easy for you to root them out. Mere crushing or suppression will not suffice. There may be again resurrection of thoughts. They should be totally eradicated, just as a loose tooth is pulled out.

When you hit at the head of a snake with a stick and crush its head, it remains absolutely motionless for some time. You think it is dead. All of a sudden it raises its head and runs swiftly. Even so the thoughts that were once crushed and suppressed by you regain strength and raise up their heads. They must be destroyed totally beyond resurrection.

It is very difficult to fix the mind on a single thought in the beginning. First diminish the number of thoughts. Try to have thoughts on one subject only. If you think of a rose you may have all sorts of thoughts connected with a rose only. You may think of different kinds of roses that are grown in different parts of the world. You may think of the various preparations that are made out of roses and their uses. You may allow even thoughts of other kinds of flowers to enter; but do not entertain thoughts of fruits and vegetables. Check the aimless wandering of the mind. Do not have thoughts at random when you think of a rose. Gradually you can fix the mind on one thought. You will have to discipline the mind daily. Eternal vigilance is needed in thought-control.

The fewer the thoughts the greater the mental strength and concentration. Suppose that the average number of thoughts that pass through your brain within one hour is one hundred. If you succeed in reducing it by constant practice of concentration and meditation to ninety you will have gained ten per cent in concentration of the mind. Every thought that is reduced adds strength and peace to the mind. Reduction of even one thought will give you mental strength and peace of mind. You may not be able to feel this in the beginning as you do not possess a subtle intellect; but there is a spiritual thermometer inside to register the reduction of even a single thought. If you reduce one thought the mental strength that you have gained by this reduction will help you to reduce the second thought easily.

In rubber plantations planters thin out the rubber trees by first cutting the small surplus trees which stand in the vicinity of big ones. By so doing they can tap more milk or rubber juice from the big trees. Even so you must think out the thoughts by destroying them one by one to drink the ambrosial milk of nectar of Immortality.

When the tail of a lizard is cut, the cut end will flutter about for some time, as there is still a little residual Prana on the tail. After one or two minutes all motion will cease. Even so, even after thinking and reduction of thoughts some thoughts will move about like the tail of the lizard. But they are powerless. They cannot do any serious havoc.

There is no vitality in them. Just as the drowning man tries to catch anything to save himself, so also these lifeless thoughts try their level best to come back to their previous state of life and vigour. If you go on with your daily practice of concentration and meditation regularly, they will die by themselves like a ghee-less lamp.

In the beginning of your practice of thought-control you will experience great difficulty. You will have to wage war with your thoughts. They will struggle their level best for their own existence. They will say, "We have every right to remain in this palace of mind. We have had a sole monopoly from time immemorial to occupy this area. Why should we vacate our dominion now? We will fight for our birthright till the end." They will pounce upon you with great ferocity. When you sit for meditation all sorts of evil thoughts will crop up. As you attempt to suppress them they will want to attack you with redoubled force and vigour. But the positive always overcomes the negative. Just as darkness cannot exist in the presence of the sun, just as a leopard cannot face a lion, so also all these dark, negative thoughts—these invisible intruders, enemies of peace—cannot stand before the sublime divine thoughts. They must die by themselves.

Just as the warrior chops off the heads of his enemies one by one, when they come out of a fortress through a trap door, so also chop up your thoughts one by one when they emerge out to the surface of the mind through the trap door of consciousness.

The substitution method is very easy and effective in the destruction of evil thoughts. Cultivate only positive virtuous thoughts of mercy, love, purity, forgiveness, integrity, generosity and humility in the garden of your mind. The negative vicious thoughts of hatred, lust, anger, greed, pride, etc., will die by themselves. It is difficult to destroy the evil thoughts by attacking them directly. You will have to tax your will and waste your energy.

Suppose the evil thoughts stay in your mind for twelve hours and recur every third day. If you can make them stay in your mind for ten hours only and recur once a week by daily practice of concentration and meditation, that would be a decided improvement. If you continue your practice the period of stay and recurrence will be gradually lessened. Eventually they will disappear altogether. Compare your present state of mind with that of last year or year before last. You will be able to find out your progress. The progress will be very slow in the beginning. It will be difficult for you to gauge your growth and advancement.

Thoughts gain strength by repetition. If you entertain an evil thought or a good thought once, this evil thought or good thought will have a tendency to recur again. Thoughts crowd together just as the birds of the same feather flock together, so also if you entertain once evil thought all sorts of evil thoughts will join together and attack you. If you entertain any good thought all good thoughts will join together.

Like attracts like. If you entertain an evil thought that thought will attract all sorts of evil thoughts from others. You will then pass on that thought to others also. A thought moves. A thought is a living dynamic force. Thought is a thing. If you allow your mind to dwell on a sublime thought this thought will attract good thoughts from others. You will pass on that good thought to others. You pollute the world with your bad thoughts. You help the world with your good thoughts.

When you reach the spiritual summit of thoughtlessness you will reach the abode of Immortality and eternal peace and supreme bliss. O Ram! start your homeward journey. March boldly in the spiritual path. Be not afraid of difficulties. Be bold. Ascend peak after peak. Cross the deep ravines of subtle Moha and pride that come on your way. Take a long jump and cross the mystic frontier of avyaktam. Kill the thoughts that wage again and again in a guerilla war. Enter now the infinite domain of pure bliss and highest knowledge. Regain your old pristine divine glory. Rest in your Sat-chit-ananda Swaroop.

4. MIND AND MEDITATION

(I)

The moment you think during meditation: "I am pure now. I do not get any evil thoughts as before" a whole battalion of evil thoughts will enter the conscious surface of the mind. But they will pass off soon. You are in the struggling stage now. A time will come when you will not entertain even a single evil thought. Meditation is a powerfull enemy of evil thoughts. The evil thoughts say: "We will be quelled soon; our host has started the meditation. Let us pounce upon the man once more." Continue your meditation vigorously. Mists and clouds cannot exist in the presence of the sun.

It is difficult to fix your mind in the beginning on the whole picture of Lord Krishna, because all the rays of the mind are not collected. Sometimes you can visualise the face, sometimes the feet, sometimes the eyes. Fix the mind on any part of the picture which the mind likes best.

The mind has attraction for certain new words or names of towns or persons. Suppose you have come across certain new words or names of towns or persons such as: 'Ecstasy,' 'Fyzabad,' 'John Herbert.' If you sit for meditation, the mind will repeat: 'Ecstasy,' 'Fyzabad,' 'John Herbert.' Sometimes it will sing some songs, repeat some old poems or Sanskrit slokas which you had learnt by heart during your boyhood. Watch the mind carefully and try to bring it back to the point or centre of meditation.

Winter is very congenial for vigorous meditation. You will not get tired even if you meditate for hours together at a stretch. But in the morning hours laziness will try its level best to overpower you. If you cover yourself up with one or two warm blankets you will feel quite comfortable. You do not like to get up in the early morning, even though the repeated alarm wakes you up again and again. You decide: "Let me sleep for fifteen minutes more and then let me start my meditation." Then you cover yourself up nicely with the blanket. You feel quite pleasant now. What is the net result? You begin to snore loudly and get up only after the sun has arisen. Days, weeks, and months will roll on like this. Every winter will pass away in this manner. Just at that time which is quite favourable for meditation. mind deceives you and overpowers you with sleep. The mind is a Master-magician. He knows several tricks and illusions. Maya operates through mind. Mysterious is the mind. Mysterious is Maya. Be alert. Be vigilant. You can control mind and Maya. Throw away the blankets as soon as you hear the alarm. Sit on Vajra Asan. Do 20 pranayams. Drowsiness will soon disappear.

When you meditate with open eyes you may see a friend in front of you and hear his voice also; but you may not be able to make out the person and his voice, because the mind is not attached to the ears or the eyes. If the mind is entirely withdrawn from the sensual objects, if the thoughts are annihilated, if likes and dislikes are destroyed, how can you perceive the world at all? You will become mindless. You will behold the Self only everywhere. All names and forms will vanish.

It is very difficult to fix the mind all at once on a point. The mind moves with a tremendous velocity. Just as a horse in a circus runs in a circle again and again, so also the mind runs in a circle again and again. Instead of allowing the mind to run in a big circle, make it run in smaller and smaller circles. Eventually it can be fixed on a point. You will have to catch hold of the mind through intelligent methods. Mere coercion and force will not do. It will make matters worse.

Sometimes you may become despondent and feel, "I have many weaknesses and defects. How can I eradicate them? How can I control this strong and impetuous mind? Will I get liberation or Nirvikalpa Samadhi in this very birth? I have not gained much even though I have practised meditation for the last 8 years". Do not be disheartened. Even if you have controlled one or two indriyas, even if you have controlled a few thoughts half the battle is won. Control of even one thought or destruction of even one Vasana will give you mental strength. Every thought that is controlled, every desire that is destroyed, every indriya that is subdued, every defect or weakness that is eradicated will add strength to the mind, will develop your will and take you one step nearer the goal. Friend! Why then lament and despair. Fight bravely on the adhyatmic battlefield. Become a spiritual soldier. Come out victorious and wear the spiritual laurels of the divine wisdom, eternal peace and supreme bliss.

(II)

Some Sadhaks do constant sadhana in a mild manner; some do intense sadhana for two hours in the morning and two hours at night. If you want to attain self-realisation quickly you must do intense and constant sadhana for a protracted period.

You may have darshan of Lord Krishna face to face. You may talk to Him also several times. You may play and eat with Him also. But if you want to have final liberation you must have Atma-sakshatkara. Nam Deva had darshan of Lord Krishna several times and yet he was declared to be a half-baked saint by the potter saint Gora Kumbhar. He had to go to Vishoba Khesar for attaining perfection or Kaivalya.

When you sit on an asan for meditation you will want to get up soon, not on account of pain in the legs but on account of impatience. Conquer this undesirable negative quality by gradually developing patience. Then you will be able to sit for three or four hours at a stretch.

During meditation you will find yourself frequently talking to somebody mentally. Stop this evil habit. Keep a careful watch over the mind.

An aspirant writes to me, "Somebody tapped at my door at 3 a.m. I woke up and opened the door. I saw Lord Krishna with crown on His head. He disappeared soon. I went through the lane in search of Him I was not able to find Him. Then I came back to my house and sat in front of my door till day-break to see Him again." Cases of somnambulists or sleep walkers are not uncommon. They dream even while standing and walking also. The above case might have been a pure case of somnambulism. You will have to be very careful in ascertaining the true nature of your spiritual experiences, whether it is a dream or an actual reality. Darshan of Lord Krishna is not so very easy. Aspirants make mistakes in the beginning.

Just as you at once remove a pebble from your shoes that troubles you, so also you must be able to remove any tormenting thought from your mind at once. Then only have you gained sufficient strength for the control of thought. Then only have you attained some real progress in the spiritual path.

An aspirant says, "I am able to meditate on one asan for three hours. In the end I become senseless but I do not fall down to the ground." If there is real meditation you will never become senseless. You will experience perfect awareness. This is a negative undesirable mental state. You will have to get over this state by perfect vigilance.

Suppose the mind runs outside during meditation forty times within one hour. If you can make it run only 38 times it is a decided improvement. You have gained some control over the mind. It demands constant practice for a long time to check such mind-wandering. Vikshep Sakti is very powerful. But sattwa is more powerful than Vikshep Sakti. Increase your sattwa and you can very easily control the oscillation of the mind.

When there is deep concentration you will experience great joy and spiritual intoxication. You will forget the body and your surroundings. All the Prana will be taken up to your head.

If you find it difficult to concentrate your mind within a room go outside and sit in an open place or terrace or by the side of a river, or in a quiet corner of a garden. You will be able to concentrate then.

When you are lying down in your bed, sometimes a big light will pass along your forehead. As soon as you try to behold the light by meditating on the sitting posture it may disappear. You may ask: "How is it that I fail to catch the light when I exert myself, whereas it comes by itself when I am lying down without an effort?" The reason is you lost the concentration as soon as you sat for meditation by entry of rajas.

Find out your centre. Dwell always in the centre. This centre is Atma or Immortal soul. This centre is the Garden of Eden. This is your original abode. This is Param Dhama. You can be above care, worry and fear now. How sweet is this home wherein there is eternal sunshine and perennial joy!

O friend! wake up! sleep no more. Meditate. It is Brahma-muhurta now! Open the gate of the temple of the Lord in your heart with the key of love. Hear the music of the soul. Sing the song of Prem to your Beloved. Play the melody of the Infinite. Melt your mind in His contemplation. Unite with Him. Immerse your self in the ocean of Love and Bliss.

(III)

When your house is on fire how daringly you re-enter the house to save your child who is sleeping in the room? Even so you must be very courageous when you tread on the spiritual path. You must be absolutely fearless. You must not have the least attachment to your body. Then only you will have self-realisation quickly. Timid people are absolutely unfit for the spiritual line.

If there are mangoes on the top of a big tree you do not jump all at once to pluck them. It is impossible. You gradually climb up the tree by catching hold of the different branches and so reach the top of the tree. Even so you cannot jump all at once to the summit of the spiritual ladder. You will have to place your feet with caution on each rung of the ladder. You will have to practise Yama, Niyama, Asan, Pranayama, Pratyahara, Dharma, and Dhyana. Then only you will reach the highest rung of the ladder of Yoga, viz., Samadhi. If you are a student of Vedanta you will have to equip yourself with the four means first. Then you will have to do Sravan, Manan and Niddhidhyasan. Then only you will attain Brahma-Sakshatkara. If you are a student of Bhakti Yoga, you will have to practise the nine modes of Bhakti, viz., Sravan, Kirtan, Smaran, Padasevan, Archanam, Vandanam, Dasyam, Sakhyam and Atma-Nivedan. Then only you will attain the state of Para-Bhakti.

If chickens and fowls run hither and thither to eat various sorts of rubbish, what does the owner of the poultry do? He gives a slight tap on their heads and throws before them some grains, to eat. Gradually they leave their dirty habit of eating filth. Even so this mind runs hither and thither to eat filthy things and enjoy the five kinds of sensual objects. Give a tap on its head and make it taste gradually the spiritual bliss by practice of the Japa and meditation.

A jivan-mukta or a Bhagwata has lustrous eyes. He has a protrusion on the top of the head and thrikute space between the two eye-brows. Whatever he says will be indelibly impressed on your mind. You cannot forget it till the end of your life. He possesses a tremendous power of attraction. He will clear all your doubts in a marvellous manner. You will enjoy a peculiar joy and peace in his presence. All your doubts will be cleared in his presence. Silence is his language. He is very compassionate and free from selfishness, anger, greed, egoism, lust and pride. He is an embodiment of truth, peace, knowledge and bliss.

It takes a long time for the charcoal to catch fire but gun powder can be ignited within the twinkling of an eye. Even so it takes a long time to ignite the fire of knowledge for a man whose heart is impure. But an aspirant with great purity of heart gets knowledge of the self within the twinkling of an eye, within the time taken to squeeze a flower by the fingers.

Maya is a very huge saw. Lust, anger, greed, delusion, pride, jealousy, hatred, egoism, etc., are the teeth of this huge saw. All worldly-minded persons are caught up in the teeth of this saw and are crushed. Those who are endowed with purity, humility, love, dispassion, devotion and enquiry are not hurt. They escape through divine grace. They pass smoothly below the saw and reach the other side of immortality.

A piece of ordinary white paper or coloured paper has no value. You throw it away. But if there is the stamp or picture of the King or Emperor on the paper (currency notes) you keep it safe in your money purse or trunk. Even so an ordinary piece of stone has no value for you. You throw it away. But if you behold the stone-murthy of Lord Krishna at Pandharpur or any other murthy in shrines you bow your head with folded hands, because there is the stamp of the Lord on the stone. The devotee super-imposes on the stone-murthy, his own beloved and all the attributes of the Lord. Image worship is very necessary for beginners.

5. CONTROL OF THE SENSES

Many aspirants fail to enter into Samadhi or Brahmic Bliss on account of restlessness of any one of the Indriyas (senses). Control of Indriyas is indispensably requisite for spiritual Sadhan.

Develop Vairag. Without Vairag and restraint of Indriyas no meditation and Samadhi is possible. Energy will leak out if Vairagya wanes. Vairag is non-attachment to sensual objects. It is a mental state.

Control the Indriyas. Through introspection find out which Indriya is troubling you and curb it ruthlessly. Give up the objects which the particular Indriya tries to grasp. Destroy the thirst for objects and sense-enjoyments. Then you will be established in Samadhi or Supreme Peace.

Discipline the Indriyas. Speak Truth. Talk little. Observe Mowna for two hours daily. Speak sweet, loving, soft words. Don't utter harsh words. Don't abuse anybody. This is the discipline of Vak Indriya, the organ of speech.

Don't go to cinemas. Don't look at ladies with lustful eyes. When you move in the streets look at the tip of the nose or big toe and walk. Don't look hither and thither. This is the discipline of the eye, the organ of sight.

Don't attend nautch parties and don't hear vulgar music. Give up musical entertainments. Don't hear worldly topics. This is the discipline of the ear, the organ of hearing.

Don't use scents. This is the discipline of the nose, the organ of smell. Give up chillies, tamarind, tea, coffee, onions, sweetmeats, etc. Give up salt and sugar for a week. Live on simple food. Fast on Ekadashi days or live on milk. This is the discipline of the tongue, the organ of taste.

Observe Brahmacharya. This is the discipline of the reproductive organ. Sleep on a hard mat. Walk bare-footed. Don't use an umbrella. This is the discipline of the skin, the organ of touch.

Fix the mind on your Ishta Devata. Bring it back again and again when it wanders and fix it on the image. This is the Sadhan for checking the wandering mind and developing concentration. By constant, regular practice, you can fix the mind steadily on God.

You may think or falsely conjecture that senses are under your control. You may be duped. All of a sudden you will become a victim or a slave. You must have not only control of one Indriya but also Param Vasyam or supreme control of all the Indriyas. THE SENSES MAY BECOME TURBULENT AT ANY TIME. REACTION MAY SET IN. Beware!

May the Lord bestow on you Vairag, Vivek and inner Spiritual strength to control the Senses and enter into Samadhi!

6. CONQUEST OF THE MIND

The mind can be controlled by Abhyasa and Vairagya. Abhyasa is constant effort to fix the mind on God or Atma. Vairagya is dispassion or non-attachment to sensual objects.

Enquire "Who am I?" Do Vichara. Do mental Japa of OM and meditate on Atma. All thoughts will die by themselves. You will rest in Sat-Chit-Ananda Atma.

Sit alone and watch the Vrittis of the mind. Be indifferent. Remain as a Sakshi. Don't identify yourself with the Vrittis. The mind will then be under your control.

Destroy the fuel of desire, and the fire of thought will be extinguished. With the annihilation of Sankalpa, the reality of Brahman will shine. Cultivate Divine qualities such as friendliness, mercy, gladness and indifference towards happiness, pain, virtue and vice. You will get peace of mind.

Don't think of the past. Don't plan for the future. Do not allow the mind to build images. Live in the solid present.

Do a thing which the mind does not want to do. Do not do a thing which the mind wants to do.

Don't try to fulfil your desires. Don't hope. Don't expect anything. Destroy the vicious desires through virtuous desires and destroy the virtuous desires also through one strong desire for liberation.

Practice of Pranayama destroys Rajas and Tamas, makes the mind steady and one-pointed.

Study of religious books, Tapas, Charity and Sat Sang with Mahatmas, Sadhus and Sanyasins overhauls worldly vicious Samskaras and paves a long way in the control of mind.

Japa of any Mantra and Upasana destroys the impurities of the mind, makes the mind inwards, induces Vairagya. helps concentration and eventually leads to control of mind and attainment of God-consciousness.

'Kalow Kesava Kirtanat'. In this Kali Yuga the easiest way for controlling the mind and attaining Moksha is Kirtan or singing the Name of the Lord.

Food has influence over the mind. Sattwic food (milk food, etc.) calms the mind. Rajasic food (meat, alcohol, etc.). excites the mind. Take Sattwic food, have Mithahara (moderation in diet).

Destroy evil habits by establishing new good habits. Control the lower instinctive mind through the higher Sattwic mind.

Constant selfless service with Atma Bhav is highly efficacious in purifying and controlling the mind.

Don't wrestle or struggle with the mind. Be regular in your concentration and meditation. May Peace, Joy, Bliss and Immortality abide in you for ever! OM Shanti!

7. THE WAY TO BLISS

God is the dispeller of ignorance, sorrow and fear. He is the bestower of Eternal Happiness. Know Him. He ever dwelleth in thee.

Cultivate a very strong faith in God. Faith is the gateway to God. Faith can work wonders.

Put your heart, mind, intellect and soul even to your smallest acts. This is the secret of success.

Be temperate in eating, drinking, sleeping, amusements and in all things.

Follow the correct principles of living. Strive for health, strength, success and God-Realisation.

Give. Give. Give. Give freely and spontaneously. Give everything. Here lies the secret of abundance.

Always act with faith and determination. Be firm in your resolve and fiery in your determination. Have an iron will.

Let by-gones be by-gones. Let the past be buried. There is a brilliant future for you. Exert. Exert. Exert.

Be always cheerful and smile away your worries. Develop your will by eradicating desires, egoism and hatred.

Sensual indulgence leads you to destruction. Renunciation leads you to Immortality.

Right thoughts produce right deeds, right actions and an admirable character. Therefore develop right thinking.

Keep the reason pure. Free yourself from egoistic notions. Destroy I-ness and Mine-ness. Attain liberation. Be free. Enjoy Bliss.

Serve. Love. Give. Restrain (the Indriyas and mind). Be good. Do good. Be kind. Be pure. Be patient.

Grow. Expand. Evolve. Destroy separateness. Mix with all. Develop Cosmic Love. Become Selfless.

Be vigilant and diligent. Watch and Pray. Fast and Meditate. Preserve. Dismiss fear, worry and anxiety.

Serve Sadhus. Have Sat Sangh. Sing the Name of the Lord. Live in seclusion for a month. Live on milk and fruits.

"Who am I? What is Samsara? What is Brahman? What is bondage? What is freedom? What is Maya? What is Avidya?" Do Vichar. Become dispassionate. Calm the mind. Have one-pointed and a balanced state of mind always.

Embrace spirituality. Practise purity. Do charity. Develop nobility. Cultivate magnanimity. Attain Divinity.

Have purification. Do concentration. Cultivate reflection. Practise meditation. Achieve perfection.

OM TAT SAT
OM SANTI SANTI SANTI